Legal First Aid

Legal First Aid
A Guide for Health Care Professionals

Anthony L. DeWitt, RRT, CRT, JD, FAARC

Attorney at Law

Bartimus, Frickelton, Robertson, and Gorney

JONES AND BARTLETT PUBLISHERS

Sudbury, Massachusetts

BOSTON   TORONTO   LONDON   SINGAPORE

World Headquarters
Jones and Bartlett Publishers
40 Tall Pine Drive
Sudbury, MA 01776
978-443-5000
info@jbpub.com
www.jbpub.com

Jones and Bartlett
    Publishers Canada
6339 Ormindale Way
Mississauga, Ontario L5V 1J2
Canada

Jones and Bartlett
    Publishers International
Barb House, Barb Mews
London W6 7PA
United Kingdom

Jones and Bartlett's books and products are available through most bookstores and online booksellers. To contact Jones and Bartlett Publishers directly, call 800-832-0034, fax 978-443-8000, or visit our website www.jbpub.com.

Substantial discounts on bulk quantities of Jones and Bartlett's publications are available to corporations, professional associations, and other qualified organizations. For details and specific discount information, contact the special sales department at Jones and Bartlett via the above contact information or send an email to specialsales@jbpub.com.

This publication is designed to provide accurate and authoritative information in regard to the Subject Matter covered. It is sold with the understanding that the publisher is not engaged in rendering legal, accounting, or other professional service. If legal advice or other expert assistance is required, the service of a competent professional person should be sought.

Production Credits
Publisher: David Cella
Acquisitions Editor: Kristine Johnson
Associate Editor: Maro Gartside
Production Manager: Julie Champagne Bolduc
Production Assistant: Jessica Steele Newfell
Senior Marketing Manager: Barb Bartoszek
Associate Marketing Manager: Lisa Gordon

Manufacturing and Inventory Control Supervisor: Amy Bacus
Composition: Forbes Mill Press
Cover Design: Timothy Dziewit
Cover Image: © Pilar Echevarria/ ShutterStock, Inc.; Utemov Alexey/ShutterStock, Inc.; Photos.com
Printing and Binding: Malloy, Inc.
Cover Printing: Malloy, Inc.

Library of Congress Cataloging-in-Publication Data
DeWitt, Anthony L.
  Legal first aid : a guide for health care professionals / Anthony L. DeWitt. — 1st ed.
    p. cm.
  Includes bibliographical references and index.
  ISBN 978-0-7637-5847-9 (pbk. : alk. paper)
  1. Medical care—Law and legislation—United States. 2. Medical personnel—United States—Handbooks, manuals, etc. I. Title.
  [DNLM: 1. Health Personnel—legislation & jurisprudence—United States—Handbooks. 2. Health Personnel—legislation & jurisprudence—United States—Outlines. 3. Malpractice—legislation & jurisprudence—United States—Handbooks. 4. Malpractice—legislation & jurisprudence—United States—Outlines. 5. Documentation—methods—United States—Handbooks. 6. Documentation--methods--United States--Outlines. 7. Liability insurance—United States—Handbooks. 8. Liability insurance—United States—Outlines. 9. Liability, Legal—United States--Handbooks. 10. Liability, Legal—United States—Outlines. W 44 AA1 D522L 2010]
  KF3821.D49 2010
  344.7303'21—dc22
                2008048847

6048

Printed in the United States of America
13 12 11 10 09   10 9 8 7 6 5 4 3 2 1

To my wife, Ginger—my own heaven-sent angel—
without whose love and belief I would be lost.

Contents

PART 3: Legal First Aid for a Criminal Law Problem 237

Acknowledgments

I acknowledge, in no particular order of importance, the many people who contributed to this book in one way or another:

Edward D. "Chip" Robertson. My mentor and friend. The chance to work for Chip has been the best thing that ever happened to me as a lawyer.

Jim Bartimus, Jim Frickleton, Steve Gorny, Mike Rader, and **Mary Winter.** My partners at Bartimus Frickleton Robertson & Gorny, for their frequent support and several great ideas.

Vern Enge. My *Advance Newsmagazines* column editor and friend. Over the last 20 years, Vern has turned bad prose into poetry, and I owe him a great debt that cannot ever be repaid.

Readers of *Advance Newsmagazines.* More than 10,000 strong, this group of professionals has asked great questions and challenged me to write material that helps them in their practice. I am indebted to them in hundreds of ways.

Kristine Johnson and **Maro Gartside.** Jones and Bartlett Publishers benefits a great deal from their hard work, and I have benefited from their careful review and thoughtful suggestions.

Introduction

Legal First Aid in an Emergency Legal Situation: An Introduction

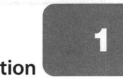

In medicine, as in almost any endeavor in life, sometimes the application of common sense and a bias for action combine to produce greater harm than had someone simply not done anything. Take, for example, the stabbing victim with the knife protruding from the chest. The helpful layperson, looking to make things better, may remove the knife with predictable consequences for the patient. A medical professional knows better than to remove the knife because the knife in place often prevents hemorrhage and complete pneumothorax. To a layperson, however, it is the knife, and not the injury, that is the problem.

The same rationale about the application of common sense applies in legal situations too. Even people who are very smart sometimes do stupid things. Often, the things that seem mandatory—like telling your side of the story—are the worst possible things you can do in a legal emergency. This chapter provides some general insight and provides some guidelines for those situations in life where you realize that you might well have a legal problem brewing.

In general, just as with first aid in a medical emergency, the sooner you find an attorney to advise and assist with a legal problem, the better the outcome will be. Although there are many legal issues you can deal with by yourself, there is almost no situation where obtaining legal counsel impairs your ability to defend yourself at a later date.

In the chapters that follow, the legal first aid outlined is set out in the order in which they should be undertaken.

◼ General Rules Regarding Legal First Aid

Employ a Family Attorney

This is not an advertisement for the truck accident attorney whose smiling face beams down at you from the interstate billboard. It is a suggestion aimed at helping ensure you have access to help in the event of a problem. Just like the flight attendant instructs you on the exits before every airplane flight, this suggestion is meant to help you in the "unlikely event" you have a serious legal problem. Before you have a legal problem is the best time to find an attorney you can trust to ask legal questions. If—before your life and life savings are at issue—you establish a relationship with an attorney, when life does throw you a curve you can deal with it. You have a family doctor; shouldn't you also have a family attorney?

Attorneys have a method by which they assist people. First, they learn as much as they can about the person and the problem, then they apply legal reasoning, precedent, statutes, and argument to assist the person in meeting their goals. Good lawyers know as much about people as they do about law and more about communication than argument. Obviously, the more a lawyer knows about you, and about the work you do, the more easily that lawyer can help you. Also, no lawyer is an expert in every legal field. If you have a problem with a commercial lease or need advice on a legal trust, a family attorney who does not practice in that area will refer you to someone who routinely handles these matters. Your lawyer is more likely to know a lawyer who can help you with a particular legal situation than you are to find one on your own or through the phone book.

Referrals are especially important when dealing with an area of the law where the attorney is unfamiliar. Civil lawyers routinely refer criminal cases to lawyers who handle those kinds of matters. But in an emergency (for example, at the police station at 10:00 p.m. on a Sunday night) any civil lawyer can do what is necessary to protect you simply by terminating questioning and invoking your right to counsel. For this reason, it is important to have someone to whom you can reach out to in an emergency.

Don't Talk About It

If something you do or don't do (or are alleged to have done or not done) could land you in legal trouble, do not talk about it with anyone other than your attorney or clergyman. Neither can be compelled in court to come forward and testify against you. Confession may be good for the soul, but it's hell on your finances.

The desire to communicate with people you respect and admire during a time of crisis is a natural human tendency. Something bad has happened to you. You feel the need to share what happened with your spouse, your significant other, your supervisor, or a close friend. It feels good to tell your side of the story to a friendly audience. They believe you, and they support you. How can anything this therapeutic be bad?

The answer is found in what lawyers call "The Hearsay Rule." If you are a party in either a civil or criminal case, what you say to others is not

hearsay. Instead, it is a "statement by a party oppo-
nent." Anyone you speak to about a matter can be
called to give testimony about what you have told
them, with certain exceptions. Doctors and health
care professionals cannot be called when the communication relates to medical treatment. Priests
(or clergy) and lawyers cannot be called to testify
against you except under very limited exceptions.
Spouses in some states have the privilege of not
testifying. But your neighbor, friend, or coworker
has no such privilege. Lawyers can ask for testimony by deposition and inquire about anything
that is reasonably likely to produce evidence. Even
questions that would never be permitted at trial
are fair game at a deposition.

More importantly, people remember and relate
things differently, particularly after the passage of
time. Have you ever played the game "telephone"
where a message is passed from one end of the
room to the other, and it changes radically from the
first person to the next person? The same thing
happens in real life every day. You may tell your
best friend that "I wasn't even in the room," but
your friend, almost 2 years later, may not recall
this. He may recall that you were in the room. An
event that is a big part of your life is a very small
part of his.

If you have a problem you should document it
right away, deal with the clinical situation, and discuss the facts of the incident only with your attorney if there is any hint that the matter could
become a lawsuit later on. Talking about the situation with friends gives the plaintiff's attorney a
chance to interview different people, find discrep-
ancies in what they remember, and paint those dis-
crepancies as lies to a jury.

Make a Record of What Happened

Although you must always satisfy your employer's demands about charting and making incident reports, to fully protect yourself you need to make an independent record of the events you believe might someday result in legal liability. You need to keep it for review by your attorney. This is why Appendix 1 is marked "Notes for My Attorney" so as to make it privileged in the eyes of the law.

The one thing that harms most defendants more than anything else is their inability to recall the facts of an incident. Although seasoned clinicians see death on a regular basis, for relatives and family members it is a singular occurrence of great importance. A jury may well assume that the inability to remember what happened is an indication that it was not important to the clinician or, worse, that the inability to remember is a cover for not telling the truth. Use Appendix 1 to record the facts of an incident and do so whenever there is a possibility that an adverse clinical outcome could wind up becoming a lawsuit.

Incident Reports

If you fill out an incident report for your employer, make sure that it records facts, not impressions, and details witnesses, not suppositions. In almost every state an incident report is protected from discovery by the plaintiff in a lawsuit. This is because the hospital should be able to rely on the candid reporting of its employees in addressing problems and fixing them. There are limited times, however, when these documents become admissible. For this reason, an incident report should be a statement of facts, not an argument that a particular person is responsible or that he or she committed an error.

In writing incident reports for employers, stick to the basics of who, what, when, and where. Unless you know for certain, omit the "how" and the "why." Incident reports should never include assumptions or unstated facts.

Be Human and Approachable

One thing that turns families off is for a clinician to act in an uncaring and unsympathetic manner. Always treat families with respect.

In interviewing hundreds of clients who came in because they were the victims of medical or hospital malpractice, almost every one has been more offended and more upset about the way they were treated (or the way their loved one was treated) than they were about the outcome of the medical misadventure. People find it difficult to sue people they like, and for this reason a good relationship with patients is often the best form of malpractice insurance.

Apologize for Outcomes, Not for Processes

Although different lawyers have different opinions, I believe that apologizing for outcomes ("I am so sorry your husband died") is appropriate and should always be done. A clinician should never apologize for the process that yielded the result.

Family members often want closure. They want to understand that they did everything they could to avoid the result that has been thrust upon them. Some families come to the hospital or emergency department with a long history of psychopathology. They may not have spoken with their loved one for months. They may have been estranged. They may be anticipating a fight over a sizable estate. Whatever the situation, family members always feel grief combined with guilt. There is always something they wish they had said after a patient dies. If you provide them with a reason, they may push that guilt off on you. So, it is OK to tell them that, like them, you are sorry for their loss. It is not OK to say anything about the process. Anything a clinician tells a family about how their patient died may later be asserted to be the cause of death in a wrongful death lawsuit. It is OK to answer questions, but do not volunteer information about medical errors or mistakes. Never admit errors. Never admit mistakes. Instead, apologize for the outcome if you must say something.

Seek Legal Help Immediately

Again, this is not an advertisement for attorneys. It is simply a suggestion to help you in the event a problem arises that your training does not prepare you to deal with. Many of us have seen the sign in our mechanic's shop that says something like:

> **Rates**
> $10/hr
> $15/hr if you watch
> $50/hr if you help

It often will be much less expensive for an attorney to assist you if you don't make more work for him or her in the beginning of the case by doing things you will come to regret later. And the only way to know where the land mines in any case are is to talk to the attorney first. Similarly, if you deal with investigators or others without understanding your rights fully, you may be intimidated into doing something you will later regret.

It is difficult for an investigator or attorney to intimidate another attorney. Lawyers know well the limits of the legal process, and so they understand when a threat is merely a threat.

Don't Be Intimidated

No state or federal agency can force you to tell your side of the story, nor can they forbid you from contacting your attorney. The only people who lose their licenses and who wind up getting thrown in jail are those who go it alone in the first instance. Often, these people are intimidated by investigators into making statements that ultimately harm their interests. Demand an attorney; say nothing else.

Buy Malpractice Insurance

If you practice as a professional, you can be sued as a professional. Malpractice insurance does not make it more likely that you will be sued. In fact, it makes it less likely that if you are sued, someone will recover against you. Insurance provides not only a fund of money to pay any judgment, but it provides you with an attorney who is there to take care of you and you alone. Malpractice insurance also often provides coverage if you are investigated by a state board. Never go it alone. If you do not have malpractice insurance today, buy it tomorrow because it is money that is very well spent. Most of us would never think of driving a car without insurance. You should never consider practicing without it either.

Practice at the State of the Art

Do not get locked into "the way we've always done it." Professional standards and research change every year. Obtain more than the minimum continuing education, and be involved in helping others learn. It keeps you up to date and helps prevent the kind of educational gaps that cause legal emergencies.

How the Legal System Works

■ Courts

There are two distinct court systems in the United States: federal and state. Federal courts are created by the constitution and by federal statutes. Federal courts usually have judges who are appointed for life, and, as a safeguard, their salaries cannot be lowered once they are in office.

- The goal of all courts is to provide speedy justice to assist persons in settling or resolving disputes.
- The purpose behind courts is to keep people from taking the law into their own hands. In the feudal system people depended on the king to settle disputes between them.
- A person goes before a court in this country to resolve a dispute between him- or herself and the other party, using judges to guide the case and juries to determine the facts.

■ Federal Courts

Courts of Limited Jurisdiction

- A federal court can only hear cases where the U.S. Congress or the Constitution makes a specific grant of jurisdiction.[1]

---

[1] Other than the Supreme Court, the Constitution does not create any courts. Congress created the federal courts and controls the reach of their jurisdiction.

- A federal court cannot hear civil cases that involve only state law issues unless the case involves citizens of different states and involves an amount of more than $75,000 and unless it is a nationwide class action.
- The federal courts also supervise the state criminal courts' adherance to basic constitutional law through a process called habeas corpus.[2]
- Federal courts handle federal criminal cases. Only crimes specified by the U.S. Code are tried in federal court.
- Some crimes, like kidnapping, are federal in nature because they involve transportation across state lines. Others involve an impact on commerce.
- Some crimes, like wire fraud, racketeering, or misuse of the mail or postal service, also involve issues only of federal law.
- When a case arises under the criminal law of the federal government, it can only be prosecuted in federal court.
- Some civil cases also arise under federal law.
- The Federal Employees Liability Act (which, for example, governs railroad workers) arose under federal law and can be tried in either state or federal court, and so can actions involving the Emergency Medical Treatment and Active Labor Act (EMTALA).
- The Racketeer Influenced Corrupt Organizations Act is a civil statute with exclusively federal jurisdiction.

---

[2] This is a writ that commands the state court to produce the prisoner's body. It was originally used to make sure states did not deprive individuals of liberty without proper process. It has now become the chief means by which death penalty cases are appealed.

- The Civil Rights Act provides for federal jurisdiction, but some states may provide greater
  protection under their laws.
- When a federal law or federal statute provides
  the basis for a right of action, federal court is an
  appropriate forum.
- When a citizen in one state sues a citizen in another state, he or she can usually sue either in
  federal or state court, depending on which one
  provides the best advantage. This is what
  lawyers call "jurisdiction based on diversity of
  citizenship."
- When citizens are from two different states,
  they are said to be diverse.
- Diversity can be the basis for a federal lawsuit
  if the amount in controversy is at least $75,000.

Removal Jurisdiction

- Even cases filed originally in state court may be
  later taken to federal court through a process
  called "removal."
- Removal is taking a case out of the state court
  and into the federal court.
- Federal courts are thought to be more favorable
  for defendants. This is not always true.

Specialized Federal Courts

Court of Claims

Whenever a person has a claim against the government or makes a claim against a government program (for example, the National Vaccine Injury
Compensation Act), the case can be filed in the U.S.
Court of Claims in Washington, DC.

Tax Court

Whenever a case involves the application of the In-
ternal Revenue Service code, a taxpayer can petition

the federal circuit courts or bring his or her action directly to the U.S. Tax Court.

Bankruptcy Courts

When people are unable to pay their bills and seek relief from their creditors, they file their case in bankruptcy court. Because bankruptcy courts involve a specialized area of the law that is provided for in the Constitution under Article II (Legislative Branch), these Bankruptcy judges are not considered federal judges with life tenure. They must be reappointed.

Administrative Agencies

- Certain administrative agencies, like the National Labor Relations Board, have the power to conduct specialized hearings in areas of law where they have written regulations.
- These hearings are administrative in nature and usually involve hearing officers and not federal judges.
- Before any of these administrative decisions can be enforced, however, a federal court must order the enforcement.

Federal Appeals Courts

- There are 12 federal circuit courts of appeal that divide the country geographically.
- The circuit courts of appeal are the primary appellate court for claims of trial court error related to cases tried in federal court.
- As an example, a federal court sitting in Mississippi is subordinate to the Fifth Circuit Court of Appeals that sits in New Orleans.
- If circuit courts of appeal reach opposite results in similar cases, the U.S. Supreme Court may exercise jurisdiction in order to resolve a "conflict" between the circuits.

Supreme Court

- The U.S. Supreme Court is the proper venue when one state sues another state.
- It is also the place where the most significant constitutional and legal questions are finally decided.
- The Supreme Court is the final arbiter of constitutional questions regarding the U.S. Constitution; the state supreme courts are the final decision-makers on issues related to their state constitutions.
- The U.S. Supreme Court cannot overturn a state court decision on state constitutional grounds (or otherwise interpret state law); it can only review cases on federal statutory or constitutional grounds.

Federal Preemption

- When Congress passes a law, it pertains only to federal issues unless the Congress specifically preempts state law.
- This preemption is based on the Supremacy Clause of the Constitution, which makes the federal law supreme over an individual state's law as long as it has a sufficient constitutional basis.

Federal Judges

- In the federal courts judges are appointed for life. The only way they can be removed is by impeachment.
- A judge in federal court does not have to retire at any certain age, which is why some Supreme Court judges are still sitting in court in their eighties.
- Federal judges cannot have their salary cut during their term in office. In other words, their salaries only go up, never down.

■ State Courts

Municipal Courts

These courts regularly handle traffic tickets and similar misdemeanor-type issues.

Magistrate or Small Claims Courts

These courts adjudicate claims involving smaller monetary amounts (usually less than $50,000 for magistrate courts and $5,000 for small claims courts).

Circuit or State District Courts

- These courts try criminal cases involving state law issues.
- They also try civil cases under state statutory or common law.
- Circuit courts (or district courts[3] in some states) hear cases either with a jury (to determine the facts) or with a judge.
- Judge-tried cases are those that involve contract matters or domestic relations matters (divorces, child custody, etc.).
- Circuit courts hold evidentiary hearings and rule on cases based on the evidence. They create a record of what they did and why so that if anyone believes they were wronged by the court's decision that person can appeal.

Courts of Appeal

- Each state has an intermediate court of appeals that exists to correct errors made by trial courts. When a court makes a mistake on the

---

[3] Where a number of counties shares a single judge, that judge is either a circuit judge (if the state breaks down by circuits) or a district judge (if the state breaks down by districts). There is little practical difference.

law or misinterprets a statute, the state court of appeals has the power to fix the error.

- The court of appeals also has the power to "supervise" lower courts by issuing writs or directives to those courts with regard to how to handle certain issues.
- Appeals courts do not hear evidence. They decide cases on the basis of the record.
- The record normally contains two sections: the paper filed by the lawyers and the testimony given by the witnesses. Appellate courts review this material to make their decisions.

State Supreme Courts

- The state supreme court is usually not a court that reviews simple trial court error. It usually hears matters of general interest and importance.
- State supreme courts usually hear matters affecting the state constitution, state revenue or tax laws, writs, and disciplinary issues involving lawyers and judges.
- Judges are normally appointed by the governor; however, some states, like Illinois and Texas, have elected supreme court judges.
- In states with elected, as opposed to appointed, judges the law tends to see-saw back and forth more because it tends to be more dominated by political concerns.

Administrative Agencies

Regulations

- The state may use administrative agencies to do what is called regulatory lawmaking.
- Regulations are written by various departments of state government and codified in the state "Code of Regulations."

- Administrative agencies not only write these regulations, they enforce them. For example:
  - The Public Service Commission might regulate utility rates by rule.
  - The Ethics Commission might regulate conduct by candidates for elected office.
  - The Finance Commission might oversee how banks and insurance companies operate.
- When the agency merely issues rules, it is operating as a rule-making body.

Judicial Functions

- When an administrative agency holds hearings and renders decisions, it is operating as a "quasi-judicial" body.
- Commissioners are not judges, and their orders, although they have the force of law, cannot be enforced without judicial review.
- When a health care practitioner is called before their state's licensing authority, the board is acting in a quasi-judicial role.
- Usually, when a board or commission makes a bad decision, that decision can be appealed through the courts and can only be enforced against a citizen by a court.

State Court Judges

- In some states judges are appointed by the governor or by a commission.
- In other states, like Texas, judges are elected by the public at large.
- Still other states have some judges that are elected and some that are appointed.
- Judges are usually responsible only to the electorate in state court. They only lose their jobs if the public votes them out or, in the rare case, where they violate the state constitution or

laws and are impeached or removed by the commission that appointed them.

Legislative Bodies

When citizens are elected to representative offices, either at the state or federal level, they become legislators, and those legislators pass legislation. Legislation is statutory lawmaking. Statutes are drafted and become law at both the state and federal level in much the same way.

Congress

Federal Law

- Congress passes federal statutes that are codified in the U.S. Code.
- There are hundreds and hundreds of pages of federal law.
- Every federal statute at some point comes before a judge for interpretation.
- How statutes are interpreted becomes a part of the federal law.
- Federal law can preempt state law.
- Article VI of the U.S. Constitution says in relevant part, "This Constitution, and the Laws of the United States which shall be made in Pursuance thereof; and all Treaties made, or which shall be made, under the authority of the United States, shall be the supreme Law of the land; and the Judges in every State shall be bound thereby, any Thing in the Constitution or Laws of any State to the Contrary notwithstanding."
- This means that where Congress wants to make a matter strictly federal in nature, it can say so in the law and the law then "preempts" state law or regulations.

- For example, the federal government has said that it will be responsible for regulating what medications are approved for human use.
- The federal law is said to "preempt" inconsistent state law.
- When a person is killed or injured by a defective drug and sues, the defendant will usually say that the case is "preempted" because a ruling by a state court that the design was defective would run counter to the federal law that says only the federal government can regulate drugs. The Supreme Court was set to decide the matter in 2008, but a decision has not yet been made.

State Legislatures

- State legislatures make state statutory law in the same way that Congress makes federal law.
- Legislators deal with both criminal and civil law issues. They may write legislation dealing with insurance and how it is sold, and they may decide to regulate how gasoline or other commodities are sold.
- They also legislate in the area of police power. They can change the definitions of crimes to meet advances in technology (like cyber-crime). They can change the penalties for crimes. They can create new crimes.
- Legislators also decide how to appropriate state money to pay for the cost of running state government by taxing the public either directly, through income taxes, or indirectly, through sales taxes.

Trials

- Trials, whether they are about medical malpractice or statutory rape, involve disputed versions of facts.

- The plaintiff (or the state in a criminal case) has the burden of proof and gets to go first. It must prove its case.
- The defendant goes last and has no burden of proof unless it assumes one (for example, suggesting that an assault was in self-defense).
- Juries (and sometimes judges) are how our legal system resolves the disputed facts.

Criminal Cases

Indictment or Information

- When the police bring in or arrest a suspect for a crime, they have the option of either charging a crime by information[4] (setting out what the state charges that the defendant did to violate the law) or by indictment (a statement by a grand jury that they believe a crime has been committed).
- If the charge is made by information, the police can arrest and jail the defendant but must hold a preliminary hearing shortly thereafter to establish to a judge probable cause to believe a crime was committed and that the defendant did it.
- An indictment is a grand jury determination that there is probable cause to charge a person with a crime.
- If there is an indictment, there does not need to be a preliminary hearing.

Preliminary Hearing

- The preliminary hearing is where the police testify to what they saw and observed and what witnesses said.

---

[4] An "information" is a pleading, just like an indictment is a pleading. It also is sometimes called a "charging document."

- Because the standard here is only probable cause—meaning that it is merely "more likely than not" that the defendant did the crime—it is rare for a defendant not to be bound over for trial.

Discovery

- In federal court the defendant has limited discovery rights and cannot usually interview witnesses.
- In state courts the defendant can sometimes interview witnesses but cannot take action that in any way seems to threaten anyone.
- In both federal and state courts, prosecutors have a duty to turn over all evidence that is potentially exculpatory such that it would aid the defense of the case.
- If the prosecutor holds back evidence, the case can and often is reversed on appeal.

Trial by Jury

- Juries are composed from the community where a case is tried, unless there is bias or prejudice against a party in that location.
- Jurors cannot have a felony conviction and must be over 18 years of age.
- Anyone who registers a car, pays taxes on a house, or registers to vote is likely to be picked as a juror.
- Jurors must take two oaths. The first is to tell the truth when the judge and lawyers ask them questions, and the second is to fairly decide the case based on the facts and the law.
- Jurors are picked from a "venire," a panel of prospective jurors.
- In most states a jury is 12 people, but in some federal cases only 6 jurors are used.

- The jurors are called into a large room and a series of questions is asked to determine if the jurors know any of the parties or witnesses or have formed any opinions about the case.
- After any jurors are excused for cause (meaning they have confessed they cannot be fair), then lawyers for both sides get to exercise something called peremptory challenges.
- These challenges allow lawyers to take people off the jury that they believe might not be sympathetic to their case.
- Jurors then hear the evidence.
- After the evidence is heard, the jury gets instructions from the judge
- After instructions, the jury selects a foreperson and begins deliberations.
- In criminal cases the jury verdict must be unanimous. If it is not, a mistrial results, and the state and defendant have to do the trial all over again.

Civil Cases

Petition or Complaint

- In a civil case the case begins with a petition or complaint that sets out the reasons why the plaintiff is suing.
- Under federal law the complaint only needs to give "notice" of the general nature of the lawsuit. Most state courts require more specific pleading.
- Usually, a defendant files both an answer and a series of motions.
- The answer is a general denial that the defendant did anything wrong.

Motions

- Defendants usually file a motion to dismiss, saying that the case cannot proceed because of one reason or another. Most of these motions are denied.

- Sometimes the defendant files a motion for more information because the plaintiff's complaint is not reasonably specific.
- Whenever one party or another wants some relief from the court about an administrative matter, it files a motion.

Discovery

- Discovery is the exchange of information between parties.
- In federal court some disclosures are mandatory and occur without any party having to file anything.
- In state court parties ask the other side to make disclosures.
- Interrogatories are used to get information about where documents are stored and who stores them.
- Document requests are used to obtain copies of documents.
- Inspection requests are used to allow people to inspect and/or photograph buildings, land, or large pieces of evidence.
- Depositions are the taking of testimony from witnesses under oath but without a judge present. Fact witnesses are often asked about what happened and when things happened in depositions. Once fact witnesses testify about what happened, "expert" witnesses may be deposed to learn about their opinions in the case.

Additional Motions

- Once facts have been discovered, there may be issues that are strictly legal that can be resolved without a jury.

- For example, if everyone agrees that the light was red, the fact is no longer disputed, and there is no "genuine issue of disputed fact" that would prevent the court from ruling strictly on the law.
- When a court rules solely on the law, the ruling is called a "summary judgment" because it does not involve a jury reaching the issues.
- Summary judgments usually benefit the defendant.

Trial

- Once the facts are known, the facts are presented to the jury.
- The jury hears the evidence and resolves the dispute about the facts.
- The judge applies the law and keeps the trial fair by including and excluding evidence based on the rules of evidence in that jurisdiction.

Jury Instructions

- One of the things the lawyers and judge discuss (and frequently argue about) is how the jury will be instructed on issues of law.
- Lawyers submit jury instructions, and the judge decides which ones to give.
- Depending on the status of the law, a judge usually gives some of the instructions the defendant asks for and some that the plaintiff requests. If an incorrect instruction is given, this may result in the case being overturned on appeal.

Additional Motions

- Once a jury reaches a verdict it provides the court with a written copy of what was decided.
- If the defendant or plaintiff disagrees, they may file a motion for a new trial.

- In some cases the defendant files a motion for judgment notwithstanding the verdict, asking the court to essentially overrule the jury.
- If the trial court believes it made an error, it can correct the error by granting a new trial. If it does not believe it made an error, then the aggrieved party can appeal.

Appeals

- Appeals may be taken to the court of appeals, to the state supreme court, or, if there is a constitutional question, to the U.S. Supreme Court.
- Only about one-tenth of 1% of cases that result in a verdict ever reach the U.S. Supreme Court. In the 2007–2008 session, the Supreme Court issued decisions in only 68 cases, a small percentage of the over 7,000 cases that were submitted (*The New York Times,* 2008).

Attorneys

Background and Education

- An attorney earns a law degree in 3 years from an approved law school.
- There is no requirement that a lawyer have any trial or courtroom experience before he or she "hangs a shingle" to practice law.
- Normally, a lawyer takes 3 to 6 years after law school to develop enough ability to be competent in court.

Practices

- Attorneys often focus their practice in a particular area if they are in a large metropolitan area because there are usually more lawyers than in rural areas.
- Attorneys in rural areas often have general practices and are pretty good at handling most general matters.
- Health law issues are almost always of a level of sophistication such that you need someone who has focused his or her practice in this area.

Experience Is Important

- You need an attorney who knows how hospitals and health care organizations operate.
- You need an attorney who will not have to learn anatomy and physiology before defending you in an action.

- However, you will seldom have only legal issues that arise in the context of health care.
- Often, you will have personal legal emergencies (e.g., car accidents, tickets, disputes with neighbors) that require an attorney's advice.
- For that reason it is a good idea to have both a private attorney for personal matters and access to a good health care law attorney.
- Just because an attorney graduated from law school doesn't make him or her competent in the area of the law where you need help.
- Attorneys are reviewed by peers in books like Martindale-Hubbell, and these books are a good place to find information on attorneys. See http://www.martindale.com for more information.

Choosing an Attorney

- If you have a family attorney, that attorney can place you into the proper hands to remedy any legal problem you have.
- If you are picking this book up for the first time because you have a legal emergency, you may be faced with picking an attorney to represent you. Below is some guidance on how to do this.

Employing a Family Attorney

- Peace of mind is valuable. A family attorney can help provide that peace of mind by being a resource to call in times of trouble.
- No lawyer is an expert in every legal field.
- If you have a problem with a legal question outside the attorney's expertise, he or she will refer you to someone who routinely handles these matters.
- Lawyers routinely make legal referrals.

- But in an emergency (for example, at the police station at 10:00 p.m. on a Sunday night) any civil lawyer (even one who doesn't do a lot of trial work) can do what is necessary to protect your rights.
- Emergencies come up when you can least afford them, making a legal relationship even more important.

Malpractice Insurance

- If you are smart enough to carry your own malpractice insurance and not unfortunate enough to believe that your employer insures you, then you have a big advantage in the selection of your lawyer.
- If you have a problem that involves your right to practice and you need legal assistance and legal advice with respect to that problem, in most cases it is covered under your malpractice policy.
- Malpractice carriers have referral and fee payment agreements with a variety of lawyers in a variety of locations. If you have a problem and you call your malpractice carrier, even if they will not pay for your consultation, they are likely to know good counsel who can assist you.

Choosing an Attorney for a Particular Case

- If you do not have an attorney, you do not have malpractice insurance, and you do not know someone you trust who can suggest one, then you have to find an attorney on your own.
- Finding an attorney requires patience and research.
- Not all attorneys are good at what they do. Not all attorneys understand what goes into defending

a health care or malpractice case. For this reason you may need to interview several before deciding on an attorney to represent you.

Research

- You need to check in Martindale-Hubbell (a listing of attorneys found in almost any library in the United States, http://www.martindale.com) to see how an attorney is rated.
- You are looking for an attorney who has the A rating for competence and the V rating for ethics. An AV-rated attorney is an attorney who is respected by his or her peers and capable of rendering excellent legal advice.
- The next step is to call the State Bar and ask if the attorney you are interested in working with has any discipline against his or her license. If the attorney has been sanctioned, disciplined, or otherwise corrected by the State Supreme Court, you may want to rethink using that attorney.
- Google is another tool that can be used to find out if the attorney has problems of any kind. News articles or reports of cases that the lawyer has been involved in may give you important clues as to the lawyer's competence.

Interview

- Once you have done some elementary background research on the lawyer, the next step is to interview the lawyer.
- For the record, the lawyer may be confused by this process. Normally, clients are interviewed by lawyers, not the other way around.
- Assert yourself! Before you disclose facts to the attorney, ask your own questions:

- Has he or she handled other cases like yours?
- What have been the results?
- How many times has he or she taken cases like yours to trial? An attorney who does not take cases to trial is likely not a strong advocate.
- How does he or she prepare for cases?
- Does he or she have expertise in discovery matters?
- Does he or she have someone to refer you to if an appeal becomes necessary?
- Will he or she be available to talk to you about the case by phone if issues arise?
- Why is research so important? Because you are bound by what your attorney does.
  - An attorney is considered an agent for the purposes of litigation.
  - That means if the attorney agrees to settle a case or agrees to stipulate to a fact, it is the same as if you agreed to do those things.
- Because you are bound by what your attorney does, you must ensure you have a thorough and competent one from the start.

Contract for Representation

- Most attorneys who do defense work bill by the hour.
- Depending on the locale, the hourly rates may be as high as $750 per hour for certain high-value lawyers.
- If you have malpractice insurance, usually the carrier takes care of paying the attorney's hourly bill.
- If you do not have insurance, the attorney will demand a retainer.

- A retainer is a reservoir of money that the lawyer maintains in his or her trust account.
- A trust account is a special account that does not draw interest. If the lawyer holds money for you, this is where he or she holds it.
- Every time the lawyer does work on your case, he or she withdraws the money from the trust account for payment.
- Normally, the retainer is for an amount that approximates how much time and effort it will take to defend the client for at least 3 months.
- Usually, there is a provision in the contract for representation that requires the client to continue to put money into the retainer as funds are drawn down out of it.
- This allows the attorney to have money on hand if he or she has to respond to an emergency motion or other matter.
- Attorneys are expensive, and this is the best reason to have your own personal policy of medical malpractice insurance.

Lawyer–Client Relationship

- You employ the lawyer; it is not the other way around.
- The attorney works for you, even if he or she is paid by an insurance company.
- The attorney must take direction on resources (that is, what experts to hire and how to spend money on the case) from the insurance company but must confer with you on the goals of representation, factual matters, and issues regarding settlement.
- The attorney offers advice and gives you direction on how to answer questions, but he or

she cannot counsel you to lie or to submit false evidence. *A lawyer who does these things should be fired and reported to the state bar.*

- Lawyers are like plumbers and electricians. They can be hired and fired at will.
- You should terminate your relationship with an attorney only when you are convinced that he or she is acting against your wishes or undermining your case.
- Keep in mind, however, that firing an attorney may make it more difficult to find another attorney to assist you with your case.

What Your Attorney Should Do

- Explain the other party's theory of the case.
- Send you a copy of everything filed in the case by any party.
- Have a full and complete understanding of the facts and the law as it pertains to your case.
- Explain the best defenses, including the witnesses that need to be interviewed and the evidence you need to give.
- Offer you advice on how to handle yourself during the period of litigation.
- Account for the time he or she spends on your case.
- Account for money he or she spends on your case (e.g., to purchase exhibits).
- Keep you updated on the progress of the case.
- Take your phone calls.
- Answer all your questions.
- Get back to you when he or she says he or she will.
- Prepare you for any depositions.
- Prepare you before any trial testimony.

- Give you his or her full loyalty and represent only you in the litigation.

What Your Attorney Should **Not** Do

- Make unauthorized disclosures of your client-confidential information.
- Counsel you to do any unlawful or improper act.
- Suggest that you remember something a certain way or that it would be better if you did. This is suborning[1] perjury and can get you both in a lot of trouble.
- Fail to communicate with you. It may be reasonable, however, to have as long as a 24-hour delay before your attorney gets back to you.
- Make decisions about settlement without advising you.

Lawyer Referral Services

- Most state bar associations operate a lawyer referral service.
- The only requirement to be on the referral service is to have a bar admission.
- Neither the bar nor a lawyer referral service warrants that any lawyer is any good at anything. They can only recommend based on what the attorney has told them.
- For this reason, just because the bar recommends a lawyer does not mean you should accept his or her representations blindly.

---

[1] To "suborn" is to encourage or permit. When a lawyer encourages a person to lie under oath or even permits it, he or she commits the crime of suborning perjury.

Lawyers Who Advertise

- The lawyer who has to advertise is generally an attorney who has more interest in finding big cases than in taking care of the clients he or she has.

- Stay away from lawyers who advertise. Generally speaking, if a lawyer has to advertise, he or she isn't that good. More importantly, a lawyer who spends a lot of time advertising and never spends time in court is acting as a referral lawyer to other lawyers.

Documentation Basics

4

What's Important and Why

Patient care documentation satisfies three purposes:

1. Documents what was done for billing purposes
2. Serves as a means of communication with other caregivers
3. Serves as a legal record of what happened in the care of the patient

Good Documentation

- Proper documentation should be aimed at satisfying all three goals.
- Documentation of routine patient care and all medications satisfies requirements for billing.
- Documenting the response to therapy, clinical parameters measured before and after treatment, observations, judgments, and communication about the patient satisfies the legal record-keeping requirements by demonstrating that the clinician acted as a reasonable and prudent practitioner.

Why Documentation Is Necessary for Legal Purposes

- Clinicians are judged by a legal standard: What would a reasonable therapist do under the same or similar circumstances? Documentation is necessary to show:
    - What the circumstances were;

- • What your reaction to the circumstances was; and
- • Whether that reaction was reasonable under the circumstances.
- Documentation preserves the record of the events and protects against memory loss caused by passage of time.
- To be admissible as an exception to hearsay rules, entries in the medical record need to be made by someone with personal knowledge at or near the time that the events occurred.
- Absent documentation there may be no way to determine if a clinician acted reasonably.
- The patient and his or her family remember what happened to them, whereas a clinician who cares for 20 people on a shift may not remember that care if it takes 2 years to file a lawsuit. Documentation is the best protection against lawsuits.

What Documentation Should Encompass

Observations

- Things a clinician sees, hears, smells, palpates, or perceives through contact with the patient
- Things the patient says
- Things family members or visitors say
- Physical findings like:
  - • Breath sounds
  - • Skin turgor
  - • Chest expansion
  - • Use of accessory muscles of ventilation
  - • Skin color (e.g., cyanosis)

Raw Clinical Data

- Pulse

- Respirations
- Pulse oximetry data
- Breath sounds
- Blood pressure readings
- Tracings
- ECG strips
- Telemetry strips
- Noninvasive blood pressure monitor printouts
- Test reports

Information Received
- Laboratory reports
- Test results from other providers
- Physician's office records (if tests were performed there)
- Calls from physicians or physician extenders (e.g., physician's assistants, advanced practice nurses)
- Statements by patients or family members

Information Communicated
- What was said
- Who said it
- When it was said

Conclusions About Data (When Appropriate)
- Evidence-based analysis that supports actions taken
- Analysis of facts that rules in or rules out courses of action

Actions Taken
- Who was there
- What was done
- When it was done
- Why it was done

- What happened after it was done
- Who the results were communicated to
- Responses to treatments or procedures
- Patient's clinical response
- Follow-up observations, actions, and treatments

Forms of Documentation

- Physician's orders
- Graphic records (e.g., temperature, pulse, and respirations)
- Narrative records
- Physician's progress notes
- Nursing notes
- Intensive care unit (ICU) clinical narrative record
- Ventilator flow sheets
- Image capture
- Medication administration reports
- Care plans
- Protocols
- Standing orders

Important Note: Incident reports are never part of the medical record and should never be referenced or referred to within the medical record. *Doing so may make them subject to discovery.*

▓ Satisfying Billing Requirements

Billing documentation should set out the type of patient care rendered.

- If the patient care is charged by time increments, the documentation should include start and stop times.
- If the patient or private insurer is billed differently for the care provided by persons giving

care, the record should indicate who gave care and for how long.

- For example, John Doe undergoes cancer surgery. His anesthesia is provided by a Certified Registered Nurse Anesthetist (CRNA) who bills for the procedure in quarter-hour increments. The CRNA is supervised by an MD anesthesiologist. Medical records should (1) document the care provided by the CRNA, (2) indicate when the MD supervised the care of the patient, (3) indicate start and stop times corresponding to quarter-hour increments, and (4) include other clinically relevant data as mandated by the standard of care.

- Usually, documentation that meets the requirements of the standard of care satisfies the requirements of billing for care.

Satisfying Communication Requirements

- Recording information in the chart is not sufficient to establish that critical information was communicated to other caregivers.

- Documentation of patient care in nursing and ancillary service charting is available information in the chart but may not be seen by other caregivers. Recording information in the chart does not relieve the clinician from notifying other caregivers about important information.

- Normally, a caregiver is responsible only for reading the information that other professionals of the same type chart.

- Doctors should read nursing and other notes but often do not.

- Prudent nurses and caregivers do not rely on physicians to obtain up-to-date information from the chart but instead provide this information orally and document it.

- For this reason it is important, whenever there is an issue that pertains to patient care, that nurses and other clinicians report information they share with other disciplines and document that sharing of information.
    - For example, Mr. French is admitted for treatment of a pulmonary disorder. He is allergic to Cipro. He tells the nurse, but physician's orders and progress notes do not reflect that the physician has been informed. No antibiotics have yet been given. Nurse writes: "Dr. Anglin called and informed of allergy to Cipro. New orders given."
- Any time information is shared orally or in writing with other caregivers, that information should be conveyed in documentation if it has the potential to affect the patient's outcome and wouldn't normally be discovered by other clinicians.
    - For example, Ben Fine is interviewed by both nurses and physicians during the admission process and is fully questioned as to other medications he is taking. The respiratory therapist assigned to do the first treatment on the patient discovers that the patient's on CPAP at home for sleep disturbance. He must communicate this to the nurse and physician and document the communication in his notes: "Patient admits that he is on CPAP machine at home. No reference to CPAP in H&P or in nursing notes. RN informed. Dr. Smith called at home and informed. No new orders."
- When patients or family provide additional or supplemental information to clinicians that is

not recorded or noted earlier, that information must be documented and the communication of that information must be documented.

- For example, Mr. Moe Fine is scheduled for surgery. Mr. Fine admits he has taken Plavix in the last 24 hours. Nurse Jones tells Dr. Smith about the Plavix. Dr. Smith tells the nurse to prep the patient for OR. Nurse Jones tells the nurse from the OR who comes to pick up the patient about the Plavix. Nurse Jones documents: "Dr. Smith informed of patient's statement that he has taken Plavix in past 24 hours. Dr. Jones instructed me to prep the patient for surgery. Report on Plavix given to OR nurse."

- If a clinician chooses to ignore information or chooses not to act on that information, documentation of the communication of the information protects the communicating clinician from a claim that he or she did not provide the information.

- Routine information that is noted by clinicians or that has no impact on patient care need not be documented but can and should be in those situations where the clinician has a suspicion that the information will be important later. Instinct and intuition should never be overlooked; if in doubt, write it out.

  - For example, Mr. Larry Fine, admitted 2 days ago for dehydration, gets morning labs that indicate his hydration status has returned to normal. Dr. Smith comments to Nurse Jones, "Larry's labs are back to normal." Jones does not need to document this information. However, if she has time and desires to, she could document, "morning laboratory results on chart wnl per Dr. Smith."

- There is a danger, however, in charting information that is normal, but only where the hospital policy is to chart by exception.
- If the hospital policy is that a clinician does not need to chart information except when that information is outside the bounds of normal readings and the clinician charts some normal information but not other normal information, the failure to document normal results may later be asserted to be a failure to detect and document abnormal information.
- Information obtained from patients and family must be documented and conflicts in information set out. Judgments about who may be correct in their reporting should not be set out.
  - For example, Mr. Fine denies the use of tobacco. Mrs. Fine denies the denial. She tells the nurse that Mr. Fine lights up in the garage every evening. This information should be documented and communicated: "Mr. Fine has denied tobacco use. Patient's wife states that he uses tobacco in the evenings. Information passed along to personal physician by phone call."
- It is not up to the clinician to decide whether the husband or the wife is right. The clinician need only report the information and make others aware of the conflict. However if other data are available (e.g., the clothes smell like cigarette smoke) that can also be documented.

▨ Essentials of Clinical Documentation

- Clinical documentation is important for billing purposes, but from a clinician's perspective its primary purpose is to create a record for you to rely on in the event someone accuses you of negligence.

- If it has all the billing requirements but does not aid your defense, it is of no use to you because it will not assist your defense at trial.
- If you skip or shortchange your clinical documentation, you are putting your reputation, license, and future on the line.
- No jury will be interested in the excuses you cite for not documenting care.
- Good documentation subscribes to certain basics. These basics will allow you to SCALP a lawyer if one comes after you and include the following:
  - Simple
    - Good documentation captures the who, what, when, how, and where of every patient interaction. Unless special circumstances exist, the "why" can usually be omitted.
    - Clinicians should use raw data whenever possible. Blood pressure of 120/60 is better than "normal blood pressure."
    - Use patient's words when reporting what patient said: "Patient states 'I can't breathe'" is better than "patient SOB."
    - Short crisp documentation is better than long narrative documentation because the more you give a lawyer to read, the more questions you will be asked in the depositions. However, brevity must be matched by accuracy and completeness.
  - Clear
    - Good documentation is clear.
    - Numbers are used where appropriate, and data are recorded in crisp and

specific terms: Avoid "tolerated well" because it is subjective, not a statement of what was done or observed. "No adverse reaction noted" means you looked for one and it wasn't there.

- Avoid vague terms, such as "seems to," "could be," and "patient might have." Document facts, stick with evidence, and do not hypothecate.
- Avoid assumptions. "Assume" is just another way to say "I was too lazy to check." If you assume and err in that assumption, a jury will assume you want to pay for it.
- Say what you mean. Do not be politically correct, but don't be insensitive either.

- Accurate
  - Gather the information that is necessary to evaluate the patient. Don't waste time getting or including irrelevant information.
  - Get the information on the right patient's chart. When information that belongs on another chart and another patient causes alterations in the treatment plan, it is a red flag for lawyers doing case review. Always make sure you're documenting on the correct chart.
  - Use only hospital-approved acronyms.
  - Make sure you record the correct time that you performed services or made observations (see "prompt" below).
- Legible
  - The best documentation in the world will not help you if it cannot be read.

Illegible documentation is hard to defend at trial.

- Legible documentation communicates to the jury that you are a careful and neat person.
- Bad handwriting that is hard to read often encourages a jury to believe you're a sloppy clinician. The lawyer on the other side can suggest that the jury take a negative view of what you wrote.
- Prompt
  - Both fish and charting begin to smell after 3 days.
  - If you want to have your documentation admitted at trial, it must be recorded at the time it happened.
  - Late entries are sometimes appropriate, however, and should be done where it is appropriate. It is better to make a late entry than not make an entry at all.

Documentation Is Guided by the Standard of Care and Hospital Policy

Documentation of clinical care should be guided by hospital policy and procedure and should correspond to the standard of care for the discipline doing the documentation. Specialty clinicians (neonatal nurses, respiratory therapists managing ventilators, etc.) may be required, by their clinical situation, to document observations and measurements that other clinicians (like physical therapists) are not required to document. Similarly, therapists may document other measurements and observations that are outside the scope of practice for nursing.

The standard of care sets forth the basics that must be documented, and the hospital policy and procedure set forth the procedure for how and when to document care. Every hospital has policies that apply to certain situations. For example, bathing, feeding, walking, weighing, and turning patients are all tasks for which a hospital publishes a policy and procedure. Most of these procedures include a guide for what should be documented. Documenting information set out in the policy meets the standard of care for the clinician. If the documentation is not sufficient, the hospital, not the clinician, bears the responsibility.

▪ In the Absence of Policy, Standard of Care Sets the Minimum Standard for Documentation

Every diagnosis, every disease state, and every condition involves a standard of care determination. Normally, that is made by the caregiver at the bedside. For example, if doing a blood gas on a patient for the first time, therapists usually do an Allen's test to determine if there is collateral circulation. The Allen's test is the standard of care. One component of documenting a first-time blood gas is to document that an Allen's test was done. At a minimum, or in the absence of policy guidance by the organization, all of the steps, measurements, and techniques that are required by the standard of care of the professional must be documented and recorded.

For example, respiratory therapists are required to measure heart rates before and after treatments. The requirement to measure heart rate and respirations is a standard of care. Whenever a therapist documents a treatment where the standard of care requires the measurement of any physical parameter, that parameter should be measured and recorded.

As another example, the standard of care, as evidenced by policies and procedures in place at the hospital, requires nurses to do postoperative vital signs every 15 minutes for the first hour after transport from the recovery room. Proper documentation includes evidence that the standard of care was met by four measurements made 15 minutes apart.

Documentation should provide evidence of the following:

- All observations required by the standard of care or hospital policy and procedure were made.
- All measurements required by the standard of care or hospital policy and procedure were made.
- All time standards set by the standard of care or by hospital policy and procedure were met.
- All changes of condition were noted and reported as required by policy, procedure, or regulation.
- All requests of and communications from the patient that have an impact on patient care should be documented.
- All evidence-based conclusions that inform or direct discretionary action by the clinician should be recorded and the basis for discretionary decisions should be set forth.

For example, Mr. Jackson requests his nurse provide him with a shot of bourbon to make it easier to swallow his pills. Nurse Jones documents: "Patient requested a glass of bourbon to take his medications with. Patient has no orders that would permit him to drink alcohol. Mr. Jackson informed he cannot have alcohol. Mr. Jackson expressed extreme displeasure about not being able to drink."

As another example, Moe Fine is 2 hours postoperative when his blood pressure falls 40 torr and he complains of being lightheaded. He can't remember what day it is, or where he is. He has had a change in his physical condition (blood pressure) and in his mentation and sensorium. This information must be recorded and communicated to appropriate clinicians immediately. "Patient's blood pressure now 90/60, down from 140/92 immediately post op. Patient disoriented to time and place. Dr. Smith paged at 11:32 a.m. Dr. Smith informed of clinical changes at 11:34 a.m. New orders received."

◼ Adverse Events

- An adverse event is an event in the care of the patient that is not planned and that results in actual, potential, or perceived harm to the patient. They include the following:
  - Falls
  - Dietary errors
  - Medication errors
  - Failures to provide care as ordered
  - Incorrect test results
  - Unnecessary testing
  - Unnecessary treatments
  - Clinical errors
  - Documentation errors
- Document the fact of all adverse events, but do not draw conclusions about the event or specify cause except as necessary to guide medical care.
- The fact of adverse events must be noted in the medical record.
- Observations made at the time of the adverse event must be recorded.

- Treatments and procedures used after the adverse event must be recorded.
- The cause of the error or the cause of any injury should not be included except as necessary to guide follow on care.
  - **Be careful:** Document observations, not conclusions.
  - For example, Nurse Jones comes in and finds Mr. Fine on the floor of his room. The bed rail is down, there is liquid on the floor near Mr. Fine's feet, and Mr. Fine has a large bump on his head.
    - Improper: Mr. Fine fell out of bed and bumped his head on the floor. He apparently slipped on some spilled water at the foot of his bed. Patient may have needed to go to the bathroom. Side rails were down when I came in.
    - Errors: This entry charts the nurse's conclusions about what happened, which could be wrong. She did not see Mr. Fine fall. Therefore the conclusion that he did is not evidence based. It includes information not relevant to his clinical care (water on floor) and includes suppositions (may have needed to go to the bathroom).
    - Proper: Mr. Fine found on floor with bruise to right side of forehead. Patient returned to bed. Neuro check completed. Head to toe assessment completed. Physician notified. New orders received.
    - Correct: This entry includes information about the observations made by the nurse and restricts information to

that clinically relevant to the patient's care.

- As another example, Mrs. Clayton has a patient-controlled analgesic (PCA) pump that, because it was improperly assembled, malfunctions and delivers an unknown dose of Mepergan. Ms. Clayton loses consciousness and becomes acidotic. She is transferred to the ICU for definitive therapy. Documentation should include the fact of the PCA error and the fact that the exact amount of medication delivered is not known. It must also include the name of the drug to guide follow on care. "Patient on PCA with Mepergan. On routine check patient is not responsive and PCA pump indicates malfunction. Reservoir of Mepergan HCl in pump appears to be exhausted, but was changed out with new bag 45 minutes ago at 13:00 by pharmacy. PCA pump does not show how much Mepergan patient received. Patient is comatose and requires mechanical ventilation. Patient transferred to ICU for definitive therapy."

- It is important to document adverse events even if there is no patient harm that results.
  - For example, patient received lunch tray at 11:30 a.m. Lunch tray included lemonade. Patient is allergic to lemons and that was noted on her admission form. "Patient given tray with lemonade. Patient allergic to lemons and called nurse to obtain other drink. Call made to dietary to flag dietary record. No lemonade ingested by patient."

- Whenever a physician's order regarding a medication is not carried out or is carried out incorrectly, it should be documented.
  - For example, Fay ordered to have 500 mg Rocephin IM but instead receives a larger dose of 1,000 mg. The nurse documents the error without calling attention to the error as such: "Patient given 1,000 mg Rocephin IM. Physician notified."
- When a medication is delayed because a patient is not on the floor or because of a procedure, it should be noted in the medication records. When the patient returns to the floor the nurse should record the times and medications given and the reason.
  - For example, "Mr. Green off floor to X-ray at 4:00 p.m. Rocephin given at 5:30 p.m. on his return."

■ Prepare Incident Reports Carefully

- Prepare reports "Dragnet-style:" Just the facts.
- Provide clear, concise information that will be used by the hospital's insurer and hospital attorneys in the defense of any litigation.
- Normally these are privileged, meaning that the plaintiff's attorney cannot see what you wrote.
- Do not assume that the incident report will remain privileged.
- Do not reference the incident report in any other documentation.
- Do not fix or assign blame to a particular person.
- Remember that incident reports are designed to help you if the case goes to trial; they are not a disciplinary tool.

◼ Prepare Employee Discipline Very Carefully

- Sometimes clinical errors must be dealt with through employee discipline.
- Employee discipline should not refer to patients by name, nor should it refer to specific incidents of conduct, except where necessary to lay the groundwork for discipline.
- A broad definition of misconduct (e.g., "failed to follow hospital policy and procedure") is better than a narrow one (e.g., "failed to give Mr. Jones medication that caused him to suffer renal failure").
- Employee discipline should stay away from broad assertions that a patient was harmed as a result of the employee misconduct. These documents can become admissible in later negligence cases brought by the patient or family.
- Good employee discipline should be brief, to the point, include the minimum information necessary to inform the employee of the error or offense, and should never draw conclusions.
    - Proper: On 6/11/2007 you were called to a patient room and asked by the nurse there to assess the patient's respiratory condition. You indicated you were busy. The nurse asked you to come as soon as possible. You waited 20 minutes. Hospital policy requires airway assessments be done within 5 minutes when requested. This written warning will go in your personnel file.
- This is good because it carefully lays out what happened, in general ways, and includes only the date and not the name of the floor or the patient. It would be difficult to get this document admitted in a particular patient's case.

- Improper: On 6/11/2007 you were assigned to 3N and were asked by Nurse Jones to come and assess patient Smith in 3437B. Mr. Smith was admitted for pneumonia, and the nurse wanted your assessment of his pulmonary condition. You told the nurse you had to do something else and would be back. By the time you wandered back to the unit the patient was in severe respiratory distress. Although you administered proper medications, the patient ultimately coded. You know that hospital policy is a 5-minute response time where there is a respiratory assessment required! If you had been there earlier, this patient might not have suffered from anoxic brain damage. Previously I gave you a verbal warning about being lazy and not coming when nurses called you. Now I'm giving you a written warning!

- This is bad because it identifies a nurse, a patient, and a unit, and now it is likely that this document could be admitted by the Smith family if they were able to discover it. In addition to stating that the therapist violated policy, it also states that the injury to the patient might have been caused by the therapist. The example above—rewritten to protect the innocent—is taken from an actual case involving an actual patient and facility.

▮ Send Interdepartmental Communications Through Quality Improvement

A memorandum from one department to another on a subject (like nurse staffing ratios, therapist coverage in the ICU, or similar matters) is subject to discovery in a lawsuit. When a manager fires off an angry memorandum to another department head, he or she creates a paper trail on that issue.

Let's suppose the nurse manager of the ICU is upset because the therapists are not providing sufficient coverage to the ICU. Her memo entitled, "Does Someone Have to Die Before You Staff the Unit Properly," becomes exhibit A in the plaintiff's case when someone does die, even if it has nothing to do with staffing.

Sending these kinds of communications and addressing these kinds of issues through the quality improvement department usually means that the communication and the discussions surrounding the communication are privileged from disclosure during discovery.

Prepare Your Own Record of Events When Warranted

- Not all staff can fill out incident reports.
- When an adverse event happens at a hospital, and it is likely to involve litigation later, employees can protect themselves by documenting what happened for their private files.
- The documentation should state at the top and bottom that it is "notes prepared in anticipation of litigation."
- The documentation should include all the information a clinician would normally put in an incident report.
- It should be dated and signed within 24 hours of the events at issue.
- It should be held in a safe deposit box and should not be shown to any other clinician.
- In the event of litigation, the notes should be given to your attorney.
- See Appendix 1.

■ Never Falsify Documentation: A Word of Caution

Everyone makes mistakes. That is why they put erasers on pencils. The best thing to do is learn from mistakes, not try to fix them after the fact. Yet, from time to time clinicians may be tempted to make changes or additions to the medical record to avoid sanctions. For example, rather than face employee discipline for not giving a treatment on time, an employee might record the wrong time or might record a treatment never given.

It is always better to accept discipline, even termination, rather than falsify a medical record. Although a late or missed treatment might get someone fired under the right circumstances, a false record can cost a license and might even incur criminal penalties.

This is the mirror image of good documentation. Just like good documentation prevents problems, false documentation creates a great deal more problems than it solves. There is no situation that can be made better by lying. And when you falsify records, you are lying. You are also playing into the hands of any plaintiff's lawyer.

If a therapist is charting a treatment on a patient whose hospital stay is being billed to Medicare or Medicaid, this is the creation of a false record. Because the record supports the billing claim of the hospital, submission of the claim creates liability under the False Claims Act for the false record. Because the claim is submitted by electronic means, it may implicate the federal wire fraud statute as well.

On top of the problems that come from submitting false claims, the State Board may issue a complaint against the provider for falsification of medical records that could result in suspension or revocation of the professional license of the clinician. This would, of course, be on top of the sanction of likely job loss from the employing hospital.

Frequently, after an adverse event clinicians try to go back and populate the medical record with information that makes them look less negligent. Although it is not falsification of a medical record when clinicians make a late entry because they remember information they failed to record, it tends to look that way to a jury. So, if after the patient has died and the family has retained a lawyer, a clinician modifies the medical record to include information he or she simply neglected to put in the record in the first place, the jury is likely to assume there is something fishy going on. Instead of working to make the clinician look less negligent, it has exactly the opposite effect.

I have been involved with cases where clinicians have written new information into the record after the medical records were already sent out to physicians' offices. So when the record is compared, the hospital's record is different from the one sent to the doctor's office immediately after a surgery. The jury is left to speculate about why the records are different. This does not help the clinician.

Resources

- *The Respiratory Therapists Legal Answer Book*, by Anthony L. DeWitt (2005).

Legal First Aid for a Civil Law Problem

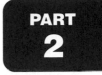

PART 2

If you have an immediate legal problem, read this section first. The best time to read this is before you have a problem. However, if you already have a problem, read this before you speak to anyone about anything (except your attorney).

Introduction and General Information

5

Recognizing a Legal Emergency

There are all kinds of legal emergencies. In health care these normally involve patients who might want to sue, employers who might want to terminate your employment, and state licensing boards who might want to take away your license for improper practice. It is important to recognize the situations where a legal emergency may present itself. What follows are general guidelines, but, in short, anything that puts your career, employment, or financial security at risk can constitute a legal emergency.

The 10 Patients (Families) to Watch Out For

1. Patients who are receiving charity care or are uninsured. These patients are not inherently bad, and including them here is not meant to suggest otherwise. But they often do have an incentive to turn the charity care they are receiving into a gold mine of a lawsuit if circumstances permit. Although, in truth, there are very few truly avaricious people out there, forewarned is forearmed.

It is said that adversity reveals genius and prosperity conceals it. This is certainly true with regard to the creative and imaginative ways that people go about using a tragedy to their own benefit. Although reputable law firms do not take cases like this, there are many out there who do. If a family seems overly interested in how much things will cost, or suggests that their loved one is receiving less care because they are poor, be alert.

2. Patients or families who lack formal education. Ignorance breeds contempt for those with higher education. It also makes it hard to admit that you don't understand what's being said. Many times a patient or family member will claim "no one told me" when, in fact, many times they were told but did not understand because the clinician used "big words." The best protection against these kinds of clients is to practice active communication skills and ask patients to repeat their understanding of what you said, and then document it.

3. Patients who make unreasonable demands. You see these patients frequently. These are the patients who want to have their evening meal at 8 p.m., want a private bath, and expect concierge services in a hospital. Although this alone does not make them suspect with regard to lawsuits, it raises suspicions because when care does not measure up to their rather high standards, they often consult a lawyer and sue. Unreasonable demands should always be documented.

4. Patients who have unreasonable expectations. It is important when dealing with patients to figure out early on what their expectations are. If they expect that their child with asthma is never going to have another attack, they are not being reasonable. When a patient has unreasonable expectations, even the best of care may not measure up. The result is often a lawsuit. Good communication by caregivers goes a long way toward preventing these problems.

5. Families with altered family dynamics. Where there are significant issues between family members or where there are family members at loggerheads over significant issues, this is where the clinician can be dragged into all-out war between factions of a family.

In one case the hospital had to step in and file a guardianship when the wife of the patient wanted something different (swift termination of life support) from what the children wanted (continuation of life support). If you honor the wishes of one group, you automatically upset the other group, often resulting in a lawsuit. This is never a good idea. However, it is better to know and be aware of the altered dynamics so that Risk Management and legal counsel can be advised and their advice and help obtained.

6. Families who write everything down and keep notes. Sometimes folks have a bad memory. Other times, people are documenting everything you do because they're planning a lawsuit. If you find people keeping records or journals, consider letting Risk Management know.

7. Families who ask, "Can I record you?" If a patient asks to make a record of your interaction, you should politely tell them no. This is also an attempt to get you to say something different from the doctor or other clinicians. If it works, the patient will claim they didn't know who to believe. Your words, in many cases taken out of context, will be used against you.

8. Patients and families who check what you tell them against what other providers tell them (e.g., "the physical therapist told me _x_, and you just told me _y_"). The family that bounces everything off every provider at some point winds up soliciting information from Housekeeping about their child's brain surgery. Never get drawn into a discussion of what some other provider told a patient. Simply stick to what you know, and do not offer other opinions. Always defer to what the doctor told them, even if you disagree. Never criticize a physician or fellow caregiver. It can have disastrous consequences for you.

9. Patients or families that do not give honest answers. When a patient is asked about history or other information and provides demonstrably false information, this is a clue that the patient cannot be trusted and should be considered a litigation risk. Consider advising Risk Management.

10. Patients or families whose reaction to bad news is "I'm gonna sue!" For obvious reasons, a patient who has this reaction is much more likely to sue than one who doesn't. Anytime you hear a threat of legal action, advise Risk Management.

■ The Unexpected Event

Within the context of how patients and family members react to medical errors and bad outcomes, it is important to understand how guilt and other human emotions play into the mix.

- Guilt is a normal human emotion.
- When loved ones die unexpectedly, family members often feel guilt at not being able to prevent it.
- In most cases that guilt stems from emotional issues left unresolved between family members.
- Where family members die unexpectedly and you hear questions like "how could you let this happen," you are seeing their guilt transferred to you in the form of blame.

▓ Misdiagnoses, Errors, and Mistakes

- As noted earlier, everyone makes mistakes.
- If you make a mistake, it does not mean you are automatically liable for all harm flowing from it.
- Similarly, if you make an error, you are not necessarily at fault.
- The judgment and discretion of a clinician are valid defenses in situations where the clinicians acted reasonably but incorrectly.

▓ You Receive a Summons, Petition, or Complaint

- If you receive notice of a lawsuit, it will come as a summons to the local circuit or district court.
- The petition (in some states) or complaint (in federal court and some states) states what the basis of the lawsuit is.
- This is a true legal emergency with deadlines. Do not wait to contact an attorney.

▓ You Receive a Call or Visit From a Board Investigator

- The State Board is not always your friend.
- Despite what they tell you, they are often not interested in the truth.
- Investigators investigate; they are paid to find facts that create reasons to discipline your license.
- If you get a phone call or a visit from an inspector or investigator, do not speak to them without an attorney present.

▓ Therefore, If:

- You have a family or patient that sets off alarm bells by their conduct; or

- You have an unexpected event that triggers defensive responses from the patient's family; or
- You make an error, misdiagnosis, or mistake; or
- You receive a summons, petition, or complaint; or
- You get a visit from the State Board

Then:

- Then you have a potential legal emergency.
- If you have such a legal emergency, the suggestions below are very important and should be followed unless an attorney advises you differently.

Silence Is Golden

- A common reaction is to talk about what happened or to try to explain your side of things. It may even seem common-sense to tell your side. But until you've talked to a lawyer, you should not say anything to anyone.
- When you give in to that "tell my side" reaction, you make it easier for someone suing you to get evidence against you.
- The only person you should speak to about a situation creating a potential legal emergency is your own personal attorney (or, in some cases, your cleric, who like your attorney, can't be subpoenaed to testify against you).
- In most situations in wanting to talk about what happened, you are reacting emotionally.
- Any statements you make, you will have to live with.
- Any statements you make, your lawyer will have to live with.

- Anything you say can and will be used against you. It is something of a "Murphy's Law" that emotional statements tend to be universally bad for your case.
- Anything you write can and will be used against you unless you mark it as notes prepared for your attorney.
- For these reasons, silence is always the best defense in a legal emergency until you have time to speak to an attorney.
- Witnesses can testify to what you said.
- Normally, a witness cannot testify to an out of court statement that was not made under oath.
- This is something that lawyers call "the hearsay rule."
- The purpose behind the rule is a witness should not testify about what someone else said if that person is available to be called as a witness.
- However, when a person is a party to litigation (meaning, one of the people suing or being sued), the hearsay rule does not apply to their statements.
- If you make an audible statement that some other witness or person can hear, they can be called to testify about that statement.
- Witnesses have bad memories that can hurt you.
  - Have you ever played the game of telephone where you start a story at one end of the room and by the time it reaches the other end of the room it is wildly different? Lawyers see this happen every day in taking witness statements. When these statements pertain to what a party or person said, the variance in the statements is often

significant. It is better for a witness to have nothing to remember than to have a witness remember something and remember it incorrectly.

- Peers and coworkers are not safe. Just because a nurse or doctor is your friend and colleague does not mean it is safe to talk to them about what happened. These individuals can be called to testify against you just as any other witness. Everything you say to them is fair game.

- Like all witnesses, memory recall degrades over time and may not be so good 2 years later when they're called to give their deposition.

Conversations with Families Should Be Witnessed

- If, after you know there is a litigation risk, you must have a conversation with a family member or patient, make sure it is witnessed.
- Ordinarily, you will not want to have such a conversation until after you seek legal advice.
- Do not get bullied into speaking before you have prepared. Remember, you're the only person who controls what you say and how you say it.

More Hazards Exist Than You Know About

- It is tempting to believe that the only thing you have to fear is a malpractice suit.
- The media spends a great deal of time on malpractice issues, but professionals get sued every day for lots of other things.
- What you tell someone about what happened may cause you trouble in one of the other areas of the law that touch on medical issues.

- *There are many other causes of action that can be advanced against you:*
  - Malpractice
    - Malpractice is the failure to use such skill and expertise as would ordinarily be used by a member of your profession under the same or similar circumstances.
    - Malpractice is usually defined by defining the standard of care for a particular professional.
    - Malpractice is proved only by expert testimony, except in the most exceptional of circumstances.
    - Malpractice is the most common form of legal liability for medical error, but it is far from the only kind of civil litigation you could be subject to.
  - Breach of fiduciary duty
    - Health care workers have fiduciary duties.
    - Legal scholars refer to the fiduciary duty as one where the professional has a duty to act in the best interests of the patient at all times.
    - A professional can breach his or her fiduciary duty by, among other things, disclosing confidential information, engaging in improper billing or treatment decisions, and other acts that do harm to the special relationship of trust.
  - HIPAA
    - HIPAA, the Health Insurance Portability and Accountability Act, imposes certain record-keeping duties on clinicians.

- Hospitals and health care entities face fines for disclosure of patient information.
- Violations are investigated by the Office of Civil Rights.
- In some cases criminal sanctions may be brought for violation of HIPAA.
- HIPAA violations may also be the basis for civil liability.

- EMTALA
  - EMTALA, the Emergency Medical Treatment and Active Labor Act, imposes liability on health care providers that fail to provide a screening examination in a medical emergency.
  - In most cases only persons who work in the emergency department fall under this Act, but the Act has been used to hold hospitals responsible for medical care rendered in an emergency on the hospital campus but outside of the emergency department.

- Battery
  - If you perform a test or procedure on a patient without informed consent, you commit the tort of Battery.
  - Battery requires informed consent and is one of the actions brought against health care providers when traditional malpractice remedies cannot be sustained.

- Fraud
  - Fraud is an intentional tort.
  - Fraud means a person made an intentional misstatement of fact to induce

another person to take some action and as a result of that action the person was damaged.

- Fraud lawsuits involving health care often center around what was told to a patient before a procedure or operation.
- Some fraud cases have involved billing patients for services not received.
- Fraud is more often than not asserted against corporations but may be asserted against individuals too.
- Slander, libel, false imprisonment, and other torts
  - Slander occurs when an untrue statement is circulated about a patient, for example, that they are an intravenous drug abuser when they are not.
  - Libel is a published statement of an untrue nature, for example, a medical record entry that a patient is an intravenous drug user when they are not.
  - False imprisonment is the tort of restraining someone's freedom of movement without just or legal cause, for example, restraining a patient who wishes to leave a medical facility who is both competent and not a hazard to him or herself or others.
- Consumer fraud
  - Certain consumer protection statutes provide a remedy against a medical provider who misrepresents or omits material facts. These "consumer fraud" cases are much harder for clinicians to defend than a classic fraud case.

- Licensure
  - The State Board can pursue licensure actions (discipline) for the following offenses, among others:
    - Theft of patient goods
    - Drug abuse, diversion, or misappropriation of drugs
    - Violations of patient privacy rights
    - Gross negligence
    - Conduct unbecoming a professional (usually convictions for violent offenses or DWI/DUI)
    - Causing patient harm
    - Breach of a professional trust or confidence
  - The State Board cases normally occur as a result of a complaint filed by a patient or employer.

▨ Legal Advice Is Critical

- *Legal advice is critical no matter what the issue.* Again, this is not an advertisement for legal services; this is simply a fact of life. If your license or your livelihood is on the line, you need a lawyer.
- Often, the thing that seems the most logical to do (e.g., telling your side of the story) is the worst thing you can do in a given set of circumstances.
- Investigators and employers often capitalize on feelings of guilt and responsibility in the hours after a tragic event as a means of facilitating either organizational or professional discipline.
- You should never talk to an investigator of any kind or a person investigating a clinical event unless and until you have conferred with counsel.

- It is critical to get legal advice before making statements and before making written records that you will be stuck with for the duration of the litigation.
- It is rarely the information that is included in a medical record that seals a defendant's fate; it is usually the information that is missing from the record.
- The sooner you get expert legal advice, the sooner you can make statements and write reports and narratives that protect your ability to work as a clinician.

Don't Hold Back When Talking to Your Lawyer

- The more your lawyer knows, the more he or she can help you.
- Some clinicians only want the lawyer to hear the good things about their story.
- Sometimes they conceal the bad facts that hurt their case. The last thing you want is to have your lawyer blindsided with bad facts. You can hurt your case by not being completely candid.
- Always err on the side of telling your lawyer everything.
- Unless you ask him or her to help you commit a crime, cover up a crime, or actively engage in fraud, what you tell your attorney can never be repeated.
- Although your attorney has an ethical duty to the court to prevent you from testifying falsely, the ethical rules prohibit his or her disclosure of client confidential communications.
- If at all possible, before you speak with your attorney, have your thoughts and ideas committed to paper for delivery to your attorney.

▓ Follow Your Lawyer's Advice

- Confucius says that many receive advice, but only the wise profit from it.
- Trust the attorney and do as he or she advises. However, this rule does not apply if your attorney advises you to lie or commit a criminal act. Although such counsel is very rare from attorneys, this is the only time you should not follow the attorney's advice.
- If you fail to follow the advice, your attorney may need to withdraw if what you do materially impairs his or her ability to assist with your case.

▓ What's Done Is Done

- You can't pour spilled milk back into the glass. What's done is done.
- Once the facts are committed to an official report or the record contains statements that harm your case, the record cannot be undone.
- You cannot lie under oath.
- Sometimes clinicians get the idea to simply rewrite the records to remove the offending data. This is lying.
- Your attorney cannot be a party to such activities.
- If your attorney knows that you have violated the law, he or she must take action to correct the situation because your attorney cannot lie to a court.
- A good attorney can explain the truth, but the best attorney in the world cannot defend someone who lies to a tribunal.

▓ Immediate Steps

If you have a legal emergency, take the following immediate steps:

- Use Appendix 1 (at the end of the book) to make a record of everything that happened.
- Do not show your notes to any person other than your attorney. Do not make copies or ask anyone to read them over.
- Use Appendix 2 to make a complete list of witnesses.
- If you have malpractice insurance, use Appendix 3 to notify your carrier of the problem.
- If you are unsure of whether there is a reason to be concerned, use the forms anyway.

The Bottom Line

- The sooner you get an attorney involved to help manage the flow of information, the better your case will be when and if you have to go to court.

Health Care Issues in Civil Law

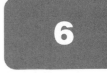

6

▪ Medical Misadventure in General

This topic deals with medical error in general and provides general guidance. If there is a specific topic in this book that deals with your situation, follow the guidance in that section. If there is not a specific topic in the book that fits your situation, refer to this portion of the text.

Overview of the Problem

When things go wrong clinically, whether it is a result of a bad outcome or someone's error, you should immediately be concerned with legal liability. Liability for medical error and medical misadventure are not limited to claims of malpractice. In recent years lawyers have been much more willing to bring claims for assault, unlawful imprisonment, and consumer fraud. Just because what happened to a patient may not be malpractice does not mean that the health care practitioner is out of the woods.

The advice that follows applies by way of illustration (but not exclusively) to the following fact situations:

- Unexpected death (especially of children)
- Irreversible hypoxic injury
- Medication errors
- Surgical errors
- Equipment errors

- Erroneous test results
- Falls
- Patient-on-patient violence

As a general rule, if there is harm that results from some preventable cause in your workplace, then you should be concerned about liability and should manage that risk.

Prevention

Medical misadventure resulting from preventable error is one of the most significant causes of injury in the United States. Recently, the U.S. Department of Health and Human Services' Centers for Medicare and Medicaid Services announced it would no longer pay for hospitalizations caused by certain errors. For this reason, prevention should always be on the minds of health care practitioners.

Risk management calls for more than simply filling out incident reports. It involves being on the lookout for dangerous situations and taking proactive measures to deal with the risks found. It involves a very active quality improvement department that views its job as preventing costly errors. Finally, it involves an overhaul of most traditional incident reporting and employee discipline systems to encourage the reporting of error and to impose discipline only for repeated or intentional violations of patient safety.

Emergency First Aid

In general:

- Document what happened in the official medical record.
- Fill out an incident report to preserve memories about what happened at the time and to name witnesses.

- If you are alleged to have done something wrong, do not give a statement to supervisors or physicians until you speak to an attorney.
- If you are not able to make your own incident report, record the results of what happened in Appendix 1 at the back of this book. Keep this form in a safe place. Do not destroy the form for at least 10 years.
- Discuss what happened only with your lawyer present. If hospital personnel or the hospital attorney want to meet to discuss matters, you should accommodate their request, but only with your attorney in attendance.
- Do not give any person a statement about the events that happened.
- Do not talk to a lawyer who represents the patient unless directed to do so by your counsel.
- Do not discuss the incident with your family members, even indirectly.
- Do not have conversations about the event in public areas.
- You may express regret over the outcome but not the process. In other words, it is OK to say "Mrs. Jones, I am sorry your husband died." It is not OK to say "I'm sorry we didn't get to the room in time to save your husband, and he died because of that."
- Even if you believe another team member made an error, do not discuss this with anyone but legal counsel. Remember, when you point one finger at someone else, there are three pointing right back at you.
- Do not discuss the events on a list-serve or through e-mail with others.
- Do not discuss the events on a public website, like MySpace.

Specific Medical Misadventures

Falls

- Document the condition of the floor and the surroundings at the time of the fall.
- Document anything the patient said or did.
- When patients say things like "this is all my fault," make sure you write it down.
- Photograph any bruising.
- Implement hospital policy with regard to falls (e.g., rendering care).
- Do not discuss the incident with family.
- File an appropriate incident report.
- Apologize for the patient's discomfort ("I am sorry that you fell"), but do not accept responsibility for the fall.

Missed Treatments

- Prepare an appropriate incident report indicating why the treatment was missed.
- If the treatment was missed because of triage, the incident report should indicate what other treatments and situations were more pressing.
- In any malpractice action, the question will be the reasonableness of the decision made by the clinician; document anything that tends to make it more reasonable that you missed the treatment (e.g., code in the emergency department, neonatal resuscitation).
- Apologize to the patient for any missed treatments ("I am sorry you were inconvenienced"), but do not accept responsibility for any error or harm that resulted.
- If harm resulted from the missed treatment (e.g., patient suffered bronchospasm for extended period), document this in the medical record and in the incident report.

- If the hospital does not permit you to make an incident report on missed treatments, prepare Appendix 1 for your own records.

Adverse Reactions to Treatments

- Document the adverse reaction.
- Document the appropriate response taken by you and other clinicians.
- If you were unaware of a patient condition like an allergy, make sure that such lack of awareness is noted in the chart (e.g., "patient never told us she was allergic to penicillin").
- Apologize for the outcome but do not accept responsibility or assume blame.
- Prepare Appendix 1 for your own records.

Equipment Malfunctions

- Identify the piece of equipment that caused the problem.
- Photograph any damage.
- Mark and tag that equipment and send it to Biomedical Engineering for analysis.
- Do not use this equipment again until cleared by Biomedical technicians
- Prepare an incident report.
- Document the specific type of problem you encountered (e.g., overheating, failure of device, fall in pressure).
- Document any patient injury.
- Under no circumstances modify or alter the equipment to make it work. Replace nonfunctional equipment. Never attempt to bypass safety devices.
- If the hospital gets sued, it may wish to sue the product manufacturer. For this reason, make sure that the equipment is preserved and not changed in the event there is ever any serious

or permanent injury (e.g., death, brain damage) that results from an equipment failure.

- Prepare Appendix 1 for your own records.

Triage

- If you have to prioritize treatments or you have to make triage decisions in an emergency, the way clinicians did during September 11, 2001, or during Hurricane Katrina, you want to document those triage decisions to the best of your ability. Your recollections may not be sufficient after the fact, particularly in a crisis.
- If the hospital has a documentation system or coding system for triage, implement it.
- It is not possible to determine who will review your actions after such an occurrence. During Katrina, health care workers were not only sued, they were tried criminally for triage decisions. Documentation is what saved the day.
- If it is not possible to write down everything that happens during triage, then every department emergency kit should have one or two small battery-powered voice recorders that clinicians can use to document their decisions in the emergency and can be used later to refresh recollections.
- Make sure that triage decisions are made in the manner approved by the hospital.
- Although documentation takes a back seat to fast action during these kinds of emergencies, it is vital to have some form of documentation available, especially where clinicians may be working 12- to 16-hour shifts every day for a week or more.
- Hospitals should always debrief their staff after such an event as part of quality assurance and preserve the record in the event of litigation.

Medication Errors

- When a patient receives an incorrect medication, it should be documented.
- Any response to the medication should be documented.
- More importantly, any "nonresponse" should be documented because patients often later claim that they had symptoms that they never had. Thus documentation to the effect that a patient did not suffer a reaction is important.
- Documentation should be aimed at any side effects that might have been expected: "Mr. Jones received Actifed tablet instead of Ativan. Patient given Ativan as ordered 30 minutes later. No adverse reactions noted from Actifed. Heart rate normal, respiratory rate normal."

Patient Violence or Patient on Patient

- Render appropriate first aid.
- Take photographs of any injuries, especially if minor.
- Document the events and what was said.
- Provide a witness statement to police if required by your employer.
- Before providing any statement to police or investigators, always consult with hospital counsel and, where applicable, your own counsel.
- Consult with counsel even if you believe everything is straightforward, because what police officers put into their reports may cause you or the facility to be sued.

Resources

- Appendix 1: Notes Prepared in Anticipation of Litigation for My Attorney.
- *The Respiratory Therapist's Legal Answer Book*, by Anthony L. DeWitt (2005).

You may find the following external resources helpful:

- Preventing Medical Injury (available online at http://www.ihi.org/IHI/Topics/PatientSafety/MedicationSystems/Literature/Preventing+medical+injury.htm).
- Institute for Health Improvement (www.ihi.org).
- Medical Errors: Tips on How to Prevent Them (available online at http://familydoctor.org/online/famdocen/home/healthy/safety/safety/736.html).
- AARP Report on Preventable Medical Injury (available online at http://www.aarp.org/research/health/carequality/Articles/aresearchimport-711-IB35.html).
- Medical Misadventure (available online at http://wrongdiagnosis.com/m/medical_misadventure/intro.htm).
- Emergency Department Visits for Medical Misadventures (abstract available online at http://gateway.nlm.nih.gov/MeetingAbstracts/102272622.html).

Documentation Failure

Overview of the Problem

Documentation failures present themselves in a number of situations. They occur, among other situations, when:

- You forget to document a treatment you gave.
- You forget to document a medication you provided.
- You provide inadequate information in your charting.
- You fail to provide proper times or data in your charting.
- A supervisor audits your work and finds errors.
- Documentation that should be in the medical record is absent.

A failure of documentation need not be a particularly difficult problem if discovered early and corrected appropriately, but it can present significant problems if not detected and remedied early.

Prevention

In a perfect world we would all have perfect recall of events and wouldn't need documentation to help us remember things. Unfortunately, very few of us have perfect recall. As a result, we require documentation.

Good documentation is a habit. Unfortunately, so is bad documentation. You prevent documentation errors by having a habit of what you document when you provide care. A routine of always providing certain information will force you to record this information every time, preventing the loss of the data.

If someone removes your charting from the medical record, and this does sometimes happen, that is not something that you can do anything about. However, if you have a routine of documenting things and you routinely document that information at all times, you can at least testify to what your normal process is at trial.

Legal First Aid

Documentation Is Missing

- If you wrote documentation of an event and it is missing, you should notify the custodian of medical records immediately. You should identify the pages that you believe are missing and what they stated. It is rare for records to have pages removed, but sometimes records do get misplaced and misfiled. If that happens and you cannot find documentation you placed in the record, you need to let someone know.
- If you discover this while reviewing records in preparation for a deposition or court proceeding, you need to alert your attorney because there could be serious evidentiary problems that require resolution.
- Do not try to re-create the records.
- If you have kept a copy of the records you might be in more trouble than you realize. Keeping a copy of the records may constitute a violation of privacy laws and regulations. However, if you

kept these records, then by all means give them to your attorney.[1]

- If you do not have a copy but you made an incident report, refer to the incident report.
- If you did not make an incident report but did make notes for your attorney in Appendix 1, then bring those to your attorney.

Documentation Is Altered

- In very rare instances documentation is not removed, but it is altered. This often takes the form of someone placing an entry on a blank line that was not there in the original. If you notice this, you should inform your attorney.
- Never alter a medical record. Never allow another employee to alter a medical record. Never allow your attorney to alter a medical record.

Documentation Does Not Provide Sufficient Data

- In some instances you will not recognize that the information you recorded is insufficient until later events make this clear. If you find that your documentation is less than adequate, you are likely stuck with it.
- Do not attempt to alter or amend the record if there has been more than 3 days elapse since the events. Although a late entry is permissible under most state laws, an entry that is weeks late (and is made only after a bad result comes to light) is usually suspect.

Medication Records Do Not Match Up

- If your hospital uses an automated record-keeping system and a drug-dispensing system,

---

[1] Your attorney may advise you to shred them, but do not do this until you have conferred with your attorney.

you may find yourself in a position where the computer shows that drugs were checked out under your name and not recorded as given by you. This can create issues with controlled substance logs and may involve a mandatory report to the professional boards. In these situations you should immediately:

- Review the charting to see if you omitted the medications and make correcting entries if possible.
- Request that the pharmacy do an audit to determine if the machine's count is correct.
- Seek legal counsel immediately.
- If your lawyer agrees, volunteer to take a blood or urine test for narcotics.[2]

You Forgot to Make an Entry

- If the error is discovered in a matter of a few hours, then make a correcting entry. If the error is discovered more than 3 days after the event, talk to your lawyer. You may wish to have your lawyer contact hospital counsel to determine if a correcting entry should be made.

Resources

- Hospital and departmental policies on documentation.
- *The Respiratory Therapists' Legal Answer Book*.
- Clinical Documentation and Compliance Manual, Health Sciences Center, University of North Texas (available online at http://www.hsc .unt.edu/policies/QuAssure/Clinical%20Docu mentation&ComplianceManual042704.pdf).

---

[2] If you have diverted these drugs or used illegal drugs, do not volunteer.

- Write It Right (online seminar available at http://www.charlydmiller.com/CLASS/document.html).
- Template-guided versus undirected written medical documentation: a prospective, randomized trial in a family medicine residency clinic, *Journal of the American Board of Family Practice* 18:464–469 (2005).
- ReDoc Documentation Software (available online at http://www.rehabdocumentation.com).

Medical Error

According to the Institute of Medicine and their 1999 report on the consequences of medical error (*To Err Is Human: Building a Safer Health System*, National Academies Press [2000]), it is both costly and commonplace in American medicine:

> Sizable numbers of Americans are harmed as a result of medical errors. Two studies of large samples of hospital admissions, one in New York using 1984 data and another in Colorado and Utah using 1992 data, found that the proportion of hospital admissions experiencing an adverse event, defined as injuries caused by medical management, were 2.9 and 3.7 percent, respectively. The proportion of adverse events attributable to errors (i.e., preventable adverse events) was 58 percent in New York, and 53 percent in Colorado and Utah.

■ Defining Medical Error

To properly deal with allegations of medical error, it is important to understand what medical error really is: An error is defined as the failure of a planned action to be completed as intended (i.e., error of execution) or the use of a wrong plan to achieve an aim (i.e., error of planning) (*To Err Is Human: Building a Safer Health System*, National Academies Press [2000]). In other words, medical error results when the plan (treat pneumonia with antibiotics) fails because (1) it is a bad plan (wrong antibiotic or diagnosis) or (2) it is a good plan (correct diagnosis) but executed poorly (wrong medications given). This is how science and medicine define medical error, and it differs slightly from what scientists call adverse events. An adverse event is an injury that flows from the way the patient's disease was managed rather than from the disease itself. So a patient who goes in for bariatric surgery and suffers a pulmonary embolus suffers an adverse event.

Importantly, from a legal perspective neither medical error nor adverse events are necessarily the basis for a lawsuit, but that often does not matter to the injured patient.

How Patients Define Error

It matters less how professionals define medical error than how patients define it. Hospital patients define medical errors much more broadly than the traditional clinical definitions of medical errors. The patient definition of medical errors includes communication problems, responsiveness, and falls, according to a new study published in the January 2007 issue of *The Joint Commission Journal on Quality and Patient Safety*. This difference is important because how a patient perceives his or her medical treatment is the single most important determinant in that patient seeking legal help for any injury that results.

When Medical Error and Adverse Events Are Not Actionable

Negligence is the failure to use that degree of skill, learning, and expertise normally used by other members of the same profession under the same or similar circumstances. Some medical error occurs in spite of clinicians using their best skill and learning.

For example, a patient who arrives in the emergency room with pulmonary edema and who claims to have been working on furniture in his garage is seen by a cardiologist who believes the most likely cause of the pulmonary edema is cardiac. He orders a cardiac catheterization, which is completely normal. Subsequent investigation reveals the man had been exposed to phosgene gas while working on PVC pipe lawn furniture with a blowtorch. The cardiologist's initial diagnosis and attempt to rule out a life-threatening cause was the principled application of skill and knowledge, but it was still incorrect. So, although it was medical error, it was not negligence.

Similarly, the bariatric surgery patient who developed a pulmonary embolus had an adverse event, but negligence only exists if the clinicians caring for him took no steps to prevent the complication (e.g., anticoagulants, compression stockings).

Prevention

The best prevention of medical error is to continually update your practice skills and continuing education. Clinicians who stay current in their field are more likely to be aware of the way medical knowledge has changed and moved forward and more likely to be practicing at the standard of care.

Legal First Aid

- How a clinician responds to a complaint about medical error depends on what the error is alleged to be, how the error is raised, and who raised it.

Allegation of Error by Patient

- If a patient alleges that you have committed an error, the most important thing to do is to avoid taking any position on the allegation. You should neither admit error nor deny it. For example:

Patient: You gave my father the wrong medicine and now he is even sicker.

Clinician: I understand you are upset that your father is sicker. I am very sorry that he is sicker, and we'll be working hard to make him better.

Patient: This is your fault.

Clinician: I understand that you feel that way. What is important is treating his condition. We are going to do everything we can to make him better.

- It is OK to say you heard the allegation. That is not an admission of its truth. It is OK to say you understand. Again, you are not agreeing. It is also important to be positive and upbeat and place a positive emphasis on things. The patient will get better. We will do all we can. These are things that even an angry patient or family member hears and wants to believe.

- Under no circumstances should you ever admit fault. You can apologize for outcomes but not for fault. An apology because the patient is sicker is not an apology because you did any thing wrong. Sometimes simply validating the patient's feelings is enough to calm the patient down.

- On the other hand, you don't want to be defensive. You don't want to say, "Nothing I did caused your father any harm." This sounds defensive, and it plays very poorly to a jury. It also puts distance between you and the people you should be trying to reach out to. Similarly, avoiding the patient and refusing to discuss the error is not helpful. You should meet, listen, and validate but not agree. Express your concerns and then explain that you have other duties and have to go. Do not get drawn into a discussion. Also be wary of patients and family members who take notes. A family member taking notes is never a good sign.

- Once a patient identifies you as being at fault, you should take all necessary measures to hand their care over to another clinician. If you do this, you will not have to have conversations like the one above. You should fill out Appendix 1 for yourself and any incident report required by your employer or insurance company. Do not discuss the error with anyone else unless compelled to do so by policy requirements (e.g., peer review committee, disciplinary meeting). If compelled, seek legal counsel first.

Allegation of Error by Hospital or Employer

- Sometimes the claim of error will arise with a coworker or an employee in another department. When that occurs first aid involves avoiding a confrontation and saying nothing. It especially precludes writing a memorandum for the record or responding to interdepartmental communications in writing. The only safe place to discuss medical error (and this is only qualifiedly safe) is in a peer review or health care quality improvement meeting.

- Under no circumstances should you ever admit error; however, you should never falsify a record or give false information to your employer or any employee tasked with investigating the incident. Admit the facts, but do not admit the conclusion that you made a medical error. You should fill out Appendix 1 for yourself, and any incident report required by your employer or insurance company. Do not discuss the error with anyone else unless compelled to do so by policy requirements (e.g., peer review committee, disciplinary meeting). If compelled, seek legal counsel first. Never make contact with patients, coworkers, or others without talking to your lawyer.

Allegation of Error by Professional Board

- Do not consent to an interview without counsel present.
- If asked to appear before the board, obtain counsel and take counsel with you to the Board meeting.

Allegation of Error in Lawsuit

- Follow the general principles laid out above. Do not speak to the patient, the family, other caregivers, or anyone else until you speak to your attorney.

Deviating From Established Protocols

From time to time there may be a question about whether it was correct or incorrect for a clinician to deviate from an accepted clinical pathway or protocol to treat a patient. Pathways and protocols cover the 95% of cases that are typical. They do not cover every situation. Sometimes, in emergency situations, it is necessary to deviate from a pathway or protocol to meet the standard of care. When this is the case, the key is documentation. If you deviate from the accepted standards laid out in a protocol or pathway, document the reasons in the medical record.

Deviating From Standards of Care

As hard as it is to believe, there are times when the standard of care would normally require you to take an action, but the patient, the patient's family, the physician, or some other agency or entity directs that you not take action that is in compliance with the standard of care. For example, a family member directs you to withhold cardiopulmonary resuscitation or rescue breathing. First, if you elect to comply with this request, you must have a reasonable basis for doing so, and you must document it. However, before complying with a request that goes against the standard of care, make sure that you both have identified the person making the request and their relationship to the patient. This is a situation where you do not want to be wrong later.

Writing Incident Reports

Most incident reports are privileged. You can lose the privilege if you refer to the report in the medical record or "incorporate" that report by reference. For this reason, mum's the word on incident reports with regard to the medical record. When you do write an incident report, remember the following:

- Only state facts you saw and heard.
- If you learned information from another party, identify the party and what they said.
- If you have to make an assumption, explain that you are making that assumption and why.
- Do not admit error.
- Do not accuse others of error in writing.
- Do not say anything you would not want on the front page of the local paper.
- Do not keep a copy for yourself. The incident report is a hospital document. If you retain a copy

for your personal information, you may actually prevent the hospital from maintaining the document's privilege. See Appendix 1.

- Do not send a copy to anyone not on the form's distribution list.

Resources

- *The Respiratory Therapists Legal Answer Book.*
- *Nurse Practitioners Business and Legal Guide.*
- *Nursing Malpractice*, by Patricia Iyer (2001).
- *Medical Malpractice Risk Management*, by James Scheper, Vicente Franklin Colon, and Nicholas Bunch (Feb. 1, 2001).
- *Nursing Malpractice: Liability and Risk Management*, by Charles C. Sharpe (May 30, 1999).
- *Nursing Negligence: Analyzing Malpractice in the Hospital Setting*, by Janet Pitts Beckmann (Mar. 20, 1996).
- *Essentials of Hospital Risk Management (Health Care Administration Series)*, by Barbara J. Youngberg (Jan. 1990).
- *Risk Management in Health Care Institutions, Second Edition: A Strategic Approach*, by Florence Kavaler (June 25, 2003).
- *Risk Management Handbook for Health Care Organizations*, by American Society for Healthcare Risk Management and Roberta Carroll (Jan. 15, 1997).
- *Clinical Risk Management: Enhancing Patient Safety*, by John Williams and Charles Vincent (Feb. 15, 2001).

Medical Privacy

At one time a violation of a patient's privacy would result in discipline, sometimes against a professional license and sometimes just from an employer. Now with the Health Insurance Portability and Accountability Act (HIPAA), medical privacy is even more important, and it is possible to violate the criminal law by violating HIPAA.

Overview

Under the common law a conversation between a physician and a patient was privileged based on the theory that only such a privilege could ensure that a physician would get the full truth from a patient and then be able to help the patient to the full extent of medical knowledge. Over time the medical privilege has extended from physicians to nurses, therapists, aides, and even hospital clerical staff.

Beginning with the advent of computerized record keeping, Congress became concerned that easy access to computerized records could result in medical privacy becoming a thing of the past. They passed HIPAA to deal with these privacy concerns.

HIPAA protects:

- Information a patient's doctors, nurses, and other health care providers put in their medical record

- Conversations a patient's doctor, nurse, or therapist has about that patient's care or treatment with other health care providers
- Information about the patient in the patient's health insurer's computer system
- Billing information about the patient at a hospital or clinic
- Most other health information about patients held by those who must follow the law

Who Must Follow the Law

- Most doctors, nurses, pharmacies, hospitals, clinics, nursing homes, and many other health care providers
- Health insurance companies, health maintenance organizations, and most employer group health plans
- Certain government programs that pay for health care, such as Medicare and Medicaid

Patients' Rights

- Ask to see and get a copy of their health records.
- Have corrections added to their health information.
- Receive a notice that tells them how their health information may be used and shared.
- Decide if they want to give their permission before their health information can be used or shared for certain purposes, such as for marketing.
- Get a report on when and why their health information was shared for certain purposes.
- And, if they believe their rights are being denied, infringed, or that their health information isn't being otherwise protected, they can

file a complaint with either their provider or health insurer or with the U.S. Government.

Penalties

The U.S. Department Health and Human Services may impose civil money penalties on a "covered entity" (usually the hospital or doctor's office) of $100 per failure to comply with a Privacy Rule requirement. That penalty may not exceed $25,000 per year for multiple violations of the identical Privacy Rule requirement in a calendar year. In addition, there are criminal penalties.

Any person who knowingly obtains or discloses individually identifiable health information in violation of HIPAA faces a fine of $50,000 and up to 1-year imprisonment. The criminal penalties increase to $100,000 and up to 5 years of imprisonment if the wrongful conduct involves false pretenses and to $250,000 and up to 10 years of imprisonment if the wrongful conduct involves the intent to sell, transfer, or use individually identifiable health information for commercial advantage, personal gain, or malicious harm. Criminal sanctions are enforced by the Department of Justice. Clinicians must take HIPAA duties very seriously.

■ Prevention

Internal Policies

The best approach to preventing privacy violations is to have in place explicit policies that are enforced with employee discipline and, if necessary, termination. These should be coupled with a very specific and proficiency-documented training program to alert clinicians of the rules and the penalties.

Prevent Surprises

People are often surprised to learn that a subpoena from a court of law does not authorize the release of protected health information. A subpoena is normally issued without a judge's order, and because it is issued by the clerk of the court instead of the judge, the rules regarding subpoenas say that they are not valid, by themselves, to authorize the release of protected health information. The best way to prevent a privacy violation based on a subpoena is to never, without prior authorization, release any information to anyone, even when presented with a subpoena. If a police officer, FBI agent, attorney, civil investigator, or Board Agent contacts you and requests that you provide information either orally or in writing regarding patient care, you should insist on seeing what is called the "Qualified Protective Order" that protects you from a violation of HIPAA.

Sometimes a lawyer's office will send out subpoenas for testimony at a deposition or trial and then say that if the documents are turned over before the deposition date no deposition will be taken. They do this to get the documents. If those documents are medical records, you cannot comply unless they can provide you with a copy of a Qualified Protective Order.

All requests for medical records of any kind should be routed to Medical Records and handled only by personnel trained to deal with these requests.

All requests for testimony should be reviewed by corporate or personal counsel, and clearance given only after a legal opinion is provided.

Effective Supervision

Every clinician, at one time or another, has slipped up and said something they should not have said in a place where they know they should not have said it. This includes elevators, lobbies, cafeterias, hallways, or even in social situations. People love to talk, and even though they recognize that medical privacy is important, some stories are just too good not to tell. The problem is, when that information gets back to the patient or, worse, to the patient's lawyer, no one will have a sense of humor about it.

Effective supervision mandates that supervisors pay attention to lunchroom talk and always take clinicians into a private area to talk about patients, patient care, or patient issues. Similarly, they must insist that staff adhere to the guidelines, and, as painful as it may be, they must further insist that if a clinician makes an error it is dealt with appropriately. If a clinician simply cannot keep his or her mouth shut, that is a clinician that no hospital or clinic needs on its staff.

Legal First Aid

- If you become aware that a document or other protected health care information has been released without authorization and you are an employee, you should contact your corporate compliance officer (CCO) for guidance. If no compliance officer exists, contact the HIPAA Privacy Officer and detail what occurred. Make good documentation of how the event occurred and what procedures were followed to release the information.

- Under no circumstances should you discuss the matter with anyone who identifies themselves as an agent of the government. Instead, contact your private or corporate counsel for guidance. This area of the law is still very new and very unsettled. Courts interpreting the guidelines have applied them differently in different jurisdictions, and, as a result, it is difficult to give broad general advice about these rules at this time. For this reason, you should:

- Contact a lawyer immediately.
- Do not speak to anyone about the problem until you talk to your lawyer.
- Make good notes about what happened and what prompted the release.
- Save all documents related to the release.

Resources

- *HIPAA for Medical Office Personnel*, by Dan Krager and Carole Krager (July 22, 2004).
- *HIPAA: Short- and Long Term Perspective on Health Care*, by Michael Doscher (June 15, 2002).
- *Ensuring a HIPAA-Compliant Informed Consent Process*, by Kimberly Irvine and Eileen Hilton (Feb. 1, 2003).
- *Getting Started with HIPAA*, by Uday O. Ali Pabrai (April 24, 2003).
- *HIPAA Transactions: A Nontechnical Business Guide for Health Care*, by Edward D. Jones III and Carolyn P. Hartley (Jan. 2004).
- *HIPAA Regulatory Documents Manual and CD: The Documents of HIPAA as a Convenient Reference in a Searchable CD-ROM for Healthcare Corporations, Hospitals, . . . and Allied Health Professionals*, by Daniel Farb (Dec. 2003).

Fiduciary Duties

A fiduciary duty arises out of a special relationship between parties. Although the dictionary defines it in a rather unhelpful way, that is where we start with an inquiry into what a breach of fiduciary duty is.

■ What Is a Fiduciary?

Webster's Unabridged Dictionary defines a fiduciary as "one that holds a fiduciary relation or acts in a fiduciary capacity to another." Going a little further, we learn that the term *fiduciary* means a relationship "premised on trust or confidence, as in the relationship between a medical clinician and a patient." Information is shared between the patient and clinician, and that information must be carefully guarded. More importantly, because the patient reposes trust in the clinician, that clinician must act for the patient's benefit, and not their own.

■ What Is a Fiduciary Relationship?

Webster's Unabridged Dictionary defines fiduciary relationship as "the relation existing when one person justifiably reposes confidence, faith, and reliance in another whose aid, advice, or protection is sought in some matter: the relation existing when good conscience requires one to act at all times for the sole benefit and interests of another with loyalty to those interests." One federal district court has stated, "Modern public policy, not the archaic whims of the common law, demands that doctors obey their implied promise of secrecy." See *Hammonds v. Aetna Casualty & Surety Co.*, 243 F.Supp. 793, 796 (N.D.Ohio 1965). Courts across the country have recognized that "[a] physician occupies a position of trust and confidence as regards his patient—a fiduciary position." See *Moore v. Webb*, 345 S.W.2d 239, 243 (Mo.App.1961); *State ex rel. Woytus v. Ryan*, 776 S.W.2d 389 (Mo.banc 1989); *State ex rel. McCloud v. Seier*, 567 S.W.2d 127, 128 (Mo. banc 1978). In other words, courts give legal importance to the promise of medical confidentiality.

◾ How Are Fiduciary Relationships Breached?

There are two ways that fiduciary relationships can be breached in a medical/clinician role. The first is by sharing privileged information in a manner that breaches the trust of the patient, and the second is by exploiting the patient for the clinician's own financial well-being.

Breach of Confidential Information

The first situation frequently arises in the context of litigation. When patients sue for personal injuries (e.g., car accident, medical negligence) they put their physical condition "at issue" in the case, meaning that any confidence they might have expected about their medical condition is waived in order for the jury to learn the extent and nature of their injuries. This waiver applies to all the matters that are of issue in the case.

Suppose Mr. Smith is in a car accident and suffers a broken back. He goes to Dr. Jones for pain management. Dr. Jones has previously treated Mr. Smith for alcoholism and depression.

Once the case is filed the defense counsel calls Dr. Jones and asks to speak to him about Mr. Smith's medical condition. The doctor agrees and tells the attorney what Mr. Smith's injuries are. Then Dr. Jones says, "He was really doing so well, having recovered from his alcoholism and depression and all."

The information about the accident is not privileged. Because the prior treatment did not bear on the issues in the case, there is a breach of a fiduciary duty by the doctor who disclosed information "outside the scope of the waiver." Dr. Jones is subject to suit, but only if Mr. Smith can prove that he was damaged by Dr. Jones' information. For purposes of this discussion, HIPAA rules and the legal obligations imposed by those rules have been ignored. For more information, see "Medical Privacy," which begins on page 98.

Self-Dealing

The problem with a breach of fiduciary relationship also arises in the context of what courts call self-dealing. If a patient is under a disability (e.g., Alzheimer's disease, dementia), a clinician cannot take advantage of it. Recently, a driver at an assisted living facility was charged with theft and endangering an adult. As part of his duties he would take residents on errands. Authorities allege that he drove the 75-year-old victim to different banks and persuaded her to withdraw money from her accounts. He took advantage of the fact that she had a medical condition that caused her to forget daily events. Only an alert teller at the bank prevented more serious losses. In this case the company that employed the driver, and of course the driver, would be liable for a breach of fiduciary duty because they exploited the vulnerable patient's trust and confidence for the driver's own personal gain.

Prevention

If you are being asked to testify in a court of law about patient issues, consult your attorney to make sure what issues are relevant to the case and what you can discuss. If you have doubts about what can be discussed, you can refuse to disclose this information and cite the medical privilege. If the court orders you to answer, as it may, you have fulfilled your duty to preserve the privilege. With regard to preventing breaches of fiduciary duty regarding employees, background checks are an important safeguard. With respect to maintaining confidentiality, see the "Medical Privacy" section earlier in this chapter.

Legal First Aid

- If you receive a subpoena, get legal assistance immediately. Find out what the issues are in the case, and testify only about those issues.
- Do not volunteer information.
- If questioned by a police officer or government agent, seek legal counsel before divulging any information. Although officers may be privileged to ask about medical matters as a part of a criminal investigation, you should not assume that they are. You should only answer such questions with counsel present.
- If you receive a notice of deposition, take it to your attorney and discuss it with him or her before you testify.
- If you are asked questions by the media, you should always answer "no comment," and direct the media person to the Press Relations or Corporate Communications office.

- If you reveal information to the press or police officers without recognizing it (for example, a private investigator in a white lab coat asks you questions, and you mistakenly assume he is a doctor), you should immediately document what happened and share that only with your attorney. If you have your own policy of malpractice insurance, you should alert your carrier.
- If you are sued for a breach of fiduciary duty, contact your attorney immediately. A breach of fiduciary duty would be covered by most medical negligence policies of insurance.

Resources

- *The Law of Fiduciary Duties*, by Rafael Chodos (Apr. 1, 2001).
- *Medical Confidentiality and Legal Privilege*, by Jean V. McHale (Kindle Edition, Mar. 14, 2007).
- *Medical Confidentiality and Crime*, by Sabine Michalowski (Dec. 2003).
- *Privacy and Confidentiality of Health Information*, by Jill Callahan Dennis (Sep. 1, 2000).

Conflict With Physicians and Nurses

▊ Overview

In nearly every setting where patients present with complex problems and multiple comorbidities, there is a disagreement about what to do, when to do it, what order to do it in, and who is in charge. This frequently creates problems for clinicians because it may not be readily discernible who really is in charge and what to do about the conflict between physicians.

Similarly, in spite of having passed the requisite licensing exams, physicians make requests that are improper, unlawful, or just plain wrong. In those instances, conflict may erupt between the clinician and the physician about whether an act can or should be taken.

Finally, it is possible in dealing with other staff members (other nurses, therapists, nurse practitioners, etc.) that interpersonal issues will eclipse the clinical issues and become a greater detriment to patient well-being than is the disease or condition that brought them into the hospital in the first place.

Prevention

In my experience about 95% of all conflicts arise out of poor communication and misunderstood motives, not real disagreements about what the proper course of action is. In most cases the best way to prevent interpersonal issues developing in the first place is to cultivate a good relationship even with the most cantankerous and unfriendly of people. This is often difficult to do, but it pays dividends when patient care is at issue.

Legal First Aid

Pure Interpersonal Conflict

- Where two clinicians disagree and do not get along they should not be assigned to work together if at all possible.
- If they must work together, they must put aside their differences.
- If they cannot put aside their differences, one or both must eventually be asked to leave.
- Interpersonal conflict presents a situation where a clinician could, in order to satisfy a need to punish someone they don't like, create a malpractice problem.
  - For example, a lab tech could create a problem for a doctor by telling a patient or family member that the doctor is unqualified or acted improperly.
  - If conflict rises to this level, it must be identified quickly and dealt with appropriately.
  - Where workers or team members are at loggerheads, some of the options include reassignment, termination, de-escalation counseling, and team-building.
  - The behavior and conflict should not be ignored; it must be remedied, and the sooner the better.
- Where conflict is based on domestic matters (e.g., girlfriends, love interests), it must be kept completely out of the workplace.

Conflict Over Patient Care Issues Creating Malpractice Concerns

There are several ways that interpersonal conflict can become malpractice issues.

- Improper orders
  - When a physician gives an order that is improper (e.g., patient allergic to drug, wrong dose, wrong route), the order should not be carried out.
  - The clinician should address the impropriety of the order through the hospital or clinic chain of command.
  - The conflict should be elevated to the level where it can be dealt with.
  - If, after using the chain of command, you are ordered to carry out an order you disagree with, you can still refuse and ask the person giving the order to carry out the order. You always have that right. Keep in mind that exercising that right may cost you your job.
  - It is far better to lose your job by being right than to lose your house by being wrong.
  - Always document your concerns and your actions.
- Conflict or error in carrying out orders
  - If an order is given and an issue arises as to whether it has been properly carried out, the best first aid is good documentation. Often, orders only appear incorrect when viewed through the lens of a retrospectoscope.
  - If an order is unclear, clarify it.
  - If an order is unusual, take steps to understand it.
  - Because orders can be confused in transcription, if a written order or a telephone

order taken by someone else appears to be incorrect ("administer 17% oxygen by mask") it is not a defense to rely on the other clinician who took the order if you are in a superior position to know the order is wrong. If conflict arises over what was said, you and the other clinician should jointly clarify the order.

- If you carry out an order that you did not realize was improperly transcribed, document your actions and identify why the order appeared to be correct.
- If you make an error carrying out an order, fill out an incident report, and use Appendix 1 from this book to make a record of events for your own counsel.
- If a clinician disagrees with your carrying out the order before you carry it out, be sure to document the conversation, and evaluate the objection even if you believe the conflict is motivated by some other source.
- Error in data analysis
  - Even the best clinicians see different data differently.
  - When a conflict arises over whether clinical data points toward one or more differing treatment options, document any disagreement in the medical record to protect yourself. If error results, fill out an incident report, and complete Appendix 1 from this book for your records to protect yourself.
  - When evaluating data, make sure you have all the data necessary.
- Conflicting orders
  - Unless hospital policy or state law dictates otherwise, the attending physician is the

person with the final say on all orders affecting a patient.

- A consultant may order tests and treatment, but if that order is countermanded by the attending physician, the attending's wishes must be respected.
- A clinician cannot opt to follow the orders of the doctor he or she likes.
- Where there is a conflict over which order to follow among competing consultants (or in the rare situation where there are multiple attending physicians), then hospital policy and the chain of command must be used to sort out the problem.
- Document any problems that arise.
- If medical error results, document the matter in an incident report and complete Appendix 1 in this book for your records.

Conflict Not Implicating Negligence

- If conflict between clinicians does not implicate patient care, it should be dealt with outside the patient care area.

Resources

- *Quick Team-Building Activities for Busy Managers: 50 Exercises That Get Results in Just 15 Minutes*, by Brian Cole Miller (Nov. 7, 2003).
- *Improving Therapeutic Communication: A Guide for Developing Effective Techniques*, by D. Corydon Hammond, Dean H. Hepworth, and Veon G. Smith (Apr. 15, 2002).
- *Civilized Assertiveness for Women: Communication with Backbone . . . not Bite*, by Judith Selee McClure (Oct. 31, 2003).
- *Managing Conflict (Lessons Learned)*, by Harvard Business School Press (Nov. 5, 2007).

- *Managing Conflict Through Communication* (3rd Edition), by Dudley D. Cahn and Ruth Anna Abigail (Mar. 9, 2006).
- *The Art of Managing Everyday Conflict: Understanding Emotions and Power Struggles*, by Erik A. Fisher and Steven W. Sharp (Apr. 30, 2004).
- *Conflict Resolution*, by Daniel Dana (Dec. 13, 2000).
- *The Art of Resolving Conflicts in the Workplace: The Six Essential Techniques with Lawrence D. Schwimmer* (Adapted from Winning Face to Face), by Lawrence D. Schwimmer and Peggy Lee Scott (1992).
- *Is That the Reason Why I Cannot Communicate Well?: Learn How to Avoid Conflict and Increase Communication Skills*, by LMFT Jef Gazley (Apr. 15, 2005).
- *Interpersonal Relationships: Professional Communication Skills for Nurses (Interpersonal Relationships)*, by Elizabeth C. Arnold and Kathleen Undeman Boggs (Nov. 15, 2002).

Conflict With Superiors

■ Overview

Conflict with superiors can present legal emergencies when those conflicts rise to the level of insubordination or other offenses for which an employer can terminate an employee. For that reason it is important to minimize, to the extent possible, conflicts with superiors.

If you develop a bad working relationship with a superior and cannot repair it, the only option may be to move to another position in another facility. Having an ongoing conflict with a superior places you in the position of not only being fired, but also being reported to your professional board.

In one case I represented a nurse who was consistently left with short staffing in an intensive care unit environment because his supervisor did not believe he needed additional help. He continually asserted that he did. Eventually, a coworker manufactured a case against him. The coworker alleged that the nurse gave Diprivan—a drug not ordered for the patient—and failed to chart it. The hospital fired him. The Board of Nursing sought to take his license. The result was, unfortunately, a trial that put the client's license on the line.

It is an unfortunate truth that when there is a conflict between a superior and a line employee, the line employee usually loses, even if there is documentary evidence that the supervisor is wrong. I represented a technician who was discharged by her supervisor for releasing confidential information. The physician and the patient both provided statements that indicated nothing had happened. The hospital took the word of the supervisor, who was not even present, instead of that of the witnesses. Because of the "employment at will" doctrine, the employee lost her job.

Prevention

There is often little you can do to prevent being harmed by a bad supervisor. If a supervisor is handling things unprofessionally or improperly, it is a good idea to document things as much as possible, but usually the best approach is simply to transfer to some other supervisor's area of responsibility or leave the employer altogether.

It is also important to know and understand your hospital's policy and its procedures. If the hospital's policy is that medications are never to be taken out of the hospital and other employees have been written up for taking medications home in their lab coat pockets, you should follow the policy and empty your pockets unless you want similar discipline.

The same is doubly true about hospital policy with regard to equipment. If the hospital forbids taking equipment home (like respirometers, compressors, etc.), then don't do it. If you routinely violate hospital policy, you routinely set yourself up for termination or discipline. Know the policies, and abide by them. This is the best protection you have because your hospital's policies, if adhered to, should protect you.

Legal First Aid

- The worst thing you can do when a supervisor attempts to discipline you is make things worse by being disrespectful or insubordinate. Therefore, if you are called to account for your conduct and you disagree, state how you disagree but do not be disrespectful.
- Never engage in physical violence. Walk away.
- Keep in mind that if you are alleged to have violated a work rule or harmed a patient, your supervisor may report you to your professional board.
- If a supervisor claims you are at fault or did something wrong, do the following:
  - Make a record of your conversation as soon after the conversation as you can.
  - Send a copy of the record to your boss with a statement that says, "If I have recorded anything improperly, please let me know so I can make the appropriate changes."
  - Know and understand your employer's policy with regard to discipline and what can and cannot be done. Often, your supervisor will not have read the policy. The policy is available in the human resources department of every employer.
  - If the event your supervisor is complaining about was witnessed by others, make note of their name and their title and where they were and what they may have heard.
  - Fill out Appendix 1 and keep it for your attorney.
  - If you are disciplined, take the discipline up through the chain of command. Take it to the highest level if you must. Even if you

are still disciplined, it will often make your superior uncomfortable enough that you won't be disciplined again.

- For more information on employee discipline, see "Employment Emergencies" below.

Resources

- *The Respiratory Therapists Legal Answer Book*, Anthony L. DeWitt (2005).
- *A Survival Guide for Working With Bad Bosses: Dealing With Bullies, Idiots, Back-Stabbers, and Other Managers from Hell*, by Gini Graham Scott (Nov. 25, 2005).
- *Nasty Bosses: How to Deal With Them Without Stooping to Their Level*, by Jay Carter (July 28, 2004).
- *Dealing With Difficult People: How to Deal with Nasty Customers, Demanding Bosses and Annoying Co-Workers*, by Roberta Cava (Aug. 14, 2006).
- *The Unfair Advantage*, by Tom Miller (June 18, 1986).
- *Self-Discipline and Emotional Control*, by Tom Miller (May 1993).
- *Winning Through Intimidation*, by Robert J. Ringer (Nov. 12, 1984).
- *To Be or Not to Be Intimidated?: That Is the Question*, by Robert J. Ringer (Feb. 25, 2004).

Employment Emergencies

▪ Overview

Of all the legal emergencies laid out in this book, this is the emergency most of my readers will face more than once and almost everyone at least once in their careers. It is the dreaded day when the boss summons you to the office and says ,"you are being accused of . . . ." If you have been fortunate enough to have avoided this day to this point in your career, count yourself lucky.

The natural tendency of most of us when we're confronted with an accusation is to not only deny it, but deny it loudly. Then we develop an attitude that often does not help us: We get defensive. There is a big difference between defending yourself and getting defensive. Getting defensive means taking things personally. It means looking for motivations in what others say It means dealing with suppositions about what might be motivating the allegations. Personalizing things never helps. Getting defensive never helps.

The keys to surviving this employment emergency are as follows:

- Remain calm.
- Get good legal counsel.
- Do not become defensive.
- Do not make the problem worse.

Prevention

The first step in preventing this kind of legal emergency is having the kind of relationship with your boss where his or her initial reaction is not to believe anything bad that is said about you. That means working hard, doing more than your fair share, and being a team player. It means not picking fights and getting along with everyone. It has often been observed that the secret to success in any business is to keep your boss's boss off your boss's back. That is certainly true when you're trying to prevent an employment emergency.

Legal First Aid

Employment emergencies arise in a variety of contexts. Below we look at some of the most common and provide some advice on what to do in each situation.

Interview by Supervisor

- If you are called into the supervisor's office to discuss your actions, you have certain rights. You should calmly and respectfully request these rights. Among the questions you should ask before you answer any questions are:
  - Who initiated this complaint?
  - When did it happen?
  - What patient does it relate to?
  - What does my charting say?
  - What do other people say happened?
  - Who else have you talked to?
- If a supervisor starts off asking you questions about an event ("Did you tell a patient that you wished they were dead?") and refuses to answer your questions about who made the complaint and what patient it relates to before asking you questions, you should simply say

that you need the information to intelligently answer the questions.

- Often, supervisors believe they can trap you in a lie, and thereby fire you more easily, if they can get you to say something that is directly contrary to what is in your charting. It is to your benefit to understand what is being said about you before you begin answering any questions about the event.
- Once you begin answering questions:
  - Don't get defensive.
  - Don't make excuses.
  - Don't talk about what mistakes other people have made.
  - Answer what you remember, but if there is charting or documentation involved, tell the person conducting the interview you need that information before you can answer effectively. After all, you treat a lot of patients in a given day, and you can't be expected to remember them all.
- When you are finished with the interview, make a record of the interview, what was said and who said it, and send a copy to your supervisor and the person who conducted the interview with a request for them to correct anything inaccurate in your recitation of events. If they fail to correct anything in your version of events, then that becomes the official record of the interview.
- If you are being investigated for anything that might reasonably be construed to violate rules of professional conduct or for which termination is a reasonable possibility, then you must contact your attorney and obtain some advice before doing anything else.

Disciplinary Action by Employer

- If an interview leads to disciplinary action, you should appeal that discipline if you are not at fault or believe you did nothing wrong.
- The hospital or employer will have a mechanism for appealing a disciplinary decision. Follow it to the letter.
- If you believe the discipline is fair and you did what you are accused of, learn from your mistake.

Termination by Employer

- Sometimes when an interview ends, it ends not with discipline (e.g., warning, reprimand, suspension) but with termination. If your employment is terminated, you should immediately contact an attorney and find out what rights you may have.
- You should take advantage of any laws that allow you to find out the cause of your termination. Some states, like Missouri, have a service letter statute that allows you to find out from your employee the true cause of your dismissal. Sometimes the true cause as recorded by the employer is completely different from what the employee is told. You can use this information later, in court, if need be.
- If you were terminated for taking action on behalf of other employees (in other words, for going to the boss and saying "all the technicians need a raise to bring them up to parity with the other hospital in town") you may have been fired in violation of the National Labor Relations Act. Contact the National Labor Relations Board (NLRB) for advice.
- If you were terminated because of the color of your skin, your race, your religion, your gender,

your pregnancy (or ability to become pregnant), or any disability, you may have a cause of action under both state and federal antidiscrimination laws. Contact your local EEOC (or state deferral agency handling human rights complaints) for additional information.

Assault by Coworker

- No employer likes fights, particularly when there are blows struck. Although it may be fair play outside the hospital to hit someone who hits you first, you should resist the urge at all costs in the health care environment. First, it violates your duty to protect patients (which includes protecting them from their bad choices). Second, no one ever sees the guy who throws the first punch.

- If you are injured by a coworker, you probably have rights under workers' compensation law if your injury is serious.

- If you are physically assaulted, you may have the right to sue for assault, battery, or other tortuous conduct.

- You may also have a right to swear out a restraining order against the offending coemployee, but keep in mind that doing so will likely cause problems for your employer. One or both of you may be terminated.

- If an assault treads into the area of sexual assault, always make a police report.

Sexual Harassment

- If you are being sexually harassed at work, you should make a report to the human resources department. Nearly every employer has a policy for stopping sexual harassment in the workplace.

- If the human resources department does not take action, contact the hospital's CCO. He or she is required to see that the hospital complies with the federal policies on sexual harassment.
- If you do not get relief from inside the hospital by following your hospital's policy on this issue, then you should seek relief from the Office of Equal Opportunity.
- Where conduct takes the form of offensive statements, those statements should be recorded on paper and the names of witnesses should be preserved.
- When the conduct takes the form of an offer to grant you a favor if you perform sexual favors, it should likewise be documented.
- A log of the dates and times of inappropriate comments and/or physical contact should be maintained.
- This information will be invaluable to your attorney and to the EEOC.
- Sexual harassment should never be tolerated, regardless of who commits it.

Sexual Harassment by Patients

From time to time patients engage in conduct that amounts to sexual harassment. This presents a serious problem for the clinician who not only has to maintain adequate clinical distance but who may be unwilling or unable to stop treating the patient. When harassed by a patient, take the following steps:

- Confront the behavior in a nonjudgmental way if possible: "Mr. Jones, I am married and I am here to offer you proper medical treatment. I cannot get involved with patients under any set of circumstances."

- If the behavior continues, tell the patient you're feeling harassed and ask them to quit: "Mr. Jones, I feel like you're making inappropriate statements to me. I am a professional, and I cannot have any kind of relationship with you. I want you to stop asking me questions dealing with sex."
- Document these conversations with precision. Use the exact words if possible.
- Report the patient to your supervisor and to nursing personnel.
- If necessary, notify the physician.
- If the patient will not stop, ask your supervisor for a different assignment. Inform the supervisor you believe this patient is creating a "hostile work environment." Explain to the supervisor why the comments are offensive. Document the conversation with your supervisor in Appendix 1 for your records.
- If the supervisor fails to take action, follow your hospital personnel policy regarding sexual harassment to the letter.

Federal Age, Sex, Race, Religion, and Disability Discrimination

- If you are being discriminated at work on the basis of race, sex, pregnancy, age, or disability, you should make a report to the human resources department. Nearly every employer has a policy for stopping discrimination in the workplace.
- If the human resources department does not take action, contact the hospital's CCO. He or she is required to see that the hospital complies with the federal policies on discrimination.
- If you do not get relief from inside the hospital by following your hospital's policy on this issue,

then you should seek relief from the Office of Equal Opportunity. The EEOC (or the state deferral agency) is charged with investigating all complaints of discrimination.

- Where conduct takes the form of offensive statements, those statements should be recorded on paper and the names of witnesses should be preserved.
- When the conduct takes the form of employee discipline or other unfavorable employment determinations (refusal to grant a promotion, leave request, etc.), the full particulars should be documented.
- A log of the dates and times of inappropriate actions should be maintained.
- This information will be invaluable to your attorney and to the EEOC.
- Discrimination should never be tolerated, regardless of who commits it.

Resources

- *The Sexual Harassment Handbook*, by Linda Gordon Howard (Feb. 15, 2007).
- *Sexual Harassment in the Workplace*, by Mary Boland (Nov. 1, 2005).
- *Sexual Harassment, Shades of Gray: Guidelines for Managers, Supervisors, and Employees*, by Susan L. Webb (May 1, 1999).
- *Age Discrimination in the American Workplace: Old at a Young Age*, by Raymond F. Gregory (Kindle Edition, Mar. 2001).
- *Harassment and Discrimination: And Other Workplace Landmines (Entrepreneur Legal Guides)*, by Gavin S. Appleby (Oct. 18, 2007).
- *The Workplace Law Advisor: From Harassment and Discrimination Policies to Hiring and Firing*

Guidelines—What Every Manager and Employee Needs to Know, by Anne Covey (Nov. 10, 2000).

- *Legal and Ethical Handbook for Ending Discrimination in the Workplace*, by David A. Robinson (July 1, 2003).
- *Lost Your Job? (Now What)*, by Terry Kohl (June 21, 2007).

Board Investigations

▓ Overview

Board investigations normally begin when an employer makes a report of an employee discharge or when a patient makes a complaint about the professional to the licensing board. When this occurs the professional board is tasked with investigating the complaint and determining if the complaint has merit.

Board investigators are rarely clinicians. Most of the time they are former police officers, detectives, or investigators. As a result they tend to see things in black and white, and they tend to care less about science and scientific reasoning. Investigators sometimes shade things in their investigations or do shoddy investigations that result in complaints being brought by the professional boards. Although this is certainly not a large number of professional investigators, there are enough to cause the average clinician to be a bit more careful when dealing with them.

If you are investigated by a professional board, you need professional legal help at the outset.

Prevention

Ideally, you have followed the steps laid out in this book when there was a complaint about your performance or patient care. Ideally, you have already made all the necessary notations and documentations both in the record and in your own notes that show what happened and when. Hopefully, you've given all this to your attorney and solicited his or her advice. Being prepared and making a record when out of the ordinary things happen is the first step at preventing the interview with the board investigator in the first place.

The second most important prevention you can have is legal representation at the very beginning of the case and from someone who has handled similar cases before. The rules in administrative hearings are different, and a lawyer should know what those rules are before he or she begins advising you.

Legal First Aid

Interview With Investigator

- If you are approached at work, agree to meet with the investigator only when your attorney can be present.
- Do not discuss the case, what happened, or anything else with the investigator.
- Do not allow a supervisor or superior to "compel" you to talk under threat of termination: They do not have the authority to force you to waive your legal rights.
- Do not succumb to threats or intimidation. The board investigator cannot put you in jail. He or she can only get angry. Tell him or her firmly (but politely) that you will not meet without your attorney, and say nothing else. Make sure to use "sir" and "ma'am" at all times. Be deferential, but do not be drawn into a discussion of any kind.

- Prepare for the meeting by reviewing your documentation (if there is any) and disclosing to your attorney everything that happened and any possible explanations for what happened.
- It is important for your attorney to know if there are individuals making the complaint who have previously expressed some desire to injure you or your reputation or get even for something they perceive you did to them.
- Let the lawyer take the lead and set the stage for the meeting.
- Do not answer any question, even one you want to answer, if the lawyer says no.
- Keep in mind that whatever you say to the investigator will be written down and only the things that help the investigator's case will be retained.
- Your attorney should make a separate record of the meeting.
- If a complaint is ultimately filed by the professional board, make sure you get it to your attorney right away.
- If you are contacted by others, including lawyers working for the hospital, do not discuss anything about the case with them.
- There is very little you can say to a board investigator to help your case, but there are lots you can say to hurt it.
- At all times maintain your calm and professional demeanor.
- Attorneys and interrogators sometimes like to push buttons to draw out reflexive or unthinking responses. Don't let your buttons get pushed.
- If anyone has to be a jerk, let it be your attorney.

Interview With Professional Board

- Sometimes the professional board will ask for a full interview with the subject of an investigation. You have a right to be represented by an attorney, and you should exercise that right.
- Again, if anyone has to be confrontational, let it be your attorney.
- Discuss only the facts, never the motivation of other people or witnesses.
- Do not discuss other unprofessional acts by other witnesses; let your attorney save that in the event of a later trial.
- Emphasize that you did what you were required to do.
- Unless you know you are at fault, do not admit fault. If you do, you are likely to be disciplined.
- Meet before the interview with your attorney and role play. Have your attorney ask you questions. Go into the meeting prepared.
- Know who is on the board and what their background is.

Minimizing Damage

- The reason there are erasers on the ends of pencils is because everyone makes mistakes. If you have made one, and you are subject to discipline for it, sometimes an attorney can help most by preventing inappropriate discipline. Professional boards always start out offering the most draconian discipline imaginable with the idea that the sanction might be negotiated downward.
- A negotiated disciplinary outcome is always better than a litigated outcome if you lose. The board has no reason to negotiate over discipline if they have won the case.

- Do not let pride guide your decisions; listen to your attorney.

Resources

- *The Respiratory Therapists Legal Answer Book.*
- *Professional Misconduct and Physician Discipline*, by the New York State Attorney General's Office (available online at http://www.health.state.ny.us/nysdoh/opmc/main.htm).

Medical Malpractice Lawsuit

▦ Overview

There are few things scarier than a 200-pound sheriff attached to a 10-page summons and petition for damages. Often, a professional will get a call to "go to personnel," and when they go they find a sheriff waiting for them, complete with gun, badge, and uniform and a piece of paper that says horrible things about the way a patient was cared for. Your initial reaction is that your professional life is over, and you're going to lose your house and car. Usually, it isn't that serious, but you can't take that for granted. It is vital that you treat this properly.

Prevention

The first best thing you can do to prevent medical malpractice lawsuits is to treat patients like people you like, even if you don't. Even if a patient is the most cantankerous, nasty, impolite whiner in the world, treat him or her like you would want someone to treat your grandfather or grandmother. You are the professional. Make it easy for the patient to like you. Make an effort to like the patient, even though they may be scared and may strike out in inappropriate ways. The best malpractice insurance in the world is for your patients to like and respect you. People do not sue people they like and respect.

The second best thing you can do is to buy a policy of malpractice insurance. Malpractice insurance does more than simply provide you with a fund of money to pay any potential judgment against you. It provides you with a lawyer to defend you against the charges. In many cases, it also provides a lawyer for a professional discipline case. This is important because this lawyer is loyal only to one client: you. He or she does not have to think about what's good for the hospital or what's good for the doctor. He or she thinks only about what is good for you. If you telling the truth helps you and hurts the doctor or hurts the hospital, your lawyer is in the best position to give you advice about what to do.

The same is not true with regard to the hospital's lawyer. Often, employees are told that the hospital has a policy of medical malpractice insurance that covers them. Technically, this is not true. The only entity or person covered by a policy insurance is the named insured, and this is the hospital. Instead, the policy simply covers the acts of the employees of the named insured, a small but significant difference. If a judgment is entered personally against you, the hospital does not have to pay it. More importantly, if the judgment is entered against the hospital and not against you, the insurer can recover some of its money by suing you for "indemnity" or "contribution" because it claims you were responsible for part of the fault. So it is very important for a hospital employee who is a professional to have their own policy of malpractice insurance.

Legal First Aid

- First and foremost, do not discuss the case with anyone but your attorney.

- Do not talk to your spouse; cases can drag on for years, people frequently get divorced, and hell hath no fury like that of a spouse scorned.
- Do not talk to your neighbors; they will remember only enough to hurt you.
- Do not talk to coworkers; they may be interested in saving their own bacon or someone else's bacon.
- Do not talk to your supervisor; their loyalty is to the employer, not to you.
- Talk to your lawyer and your cleric only.
- Contact your medical malpractice insurer and get an attorney assigned. Make an appointment as soon as possible. Do not discuss the case with anyone until you can talk to your attorney.
- Confession may be good for the soul, but it's bad for the bank account. If you believe you have to tell someone or discuss this with someone, select a licensed counselor, cleric, or attorney to talk to about it. None of these people can be called to testify about what you told them, and when you are feeling bad, you tend to say things you will later regret.
- Bring in all your documents, including your Appendix 1. Also bring:
  - Any incident reports written that pertain to the case, if the hospital gives you permission
  - Any hospital policies and procedures that apply
  - Any clinical journal articles, books, treatises, or other written documentation that supports what you did
  - A copy of the medical records in the case, if the hospital permits it
- If you did not create an Appendix 1 at the time when the events took place, you need to prepare

a narrative of what happened. Before you go in, on a piece of paper marked "Notes Prepared for My Attorney" make sure you include everything you can remember about what happened.

- Start from the beginning of the shift until the end of the shift.
- Include any other important facts, like if other employees were absent, you were working short-handed, you had the flu, and so on.
- Indicate if there were incident reports made.
- Make sure you detail all the witnesses, even people like housekeepers and dietary workers who you might not think of. Every witness must be interviewed.
- Go over your narrative as many times as possible. You want it as accurate as possible.
- On the notes, prepare a timeline of the significant events so that the attorney can see what you did and when you did it in graphic form.
- Do not rely on information from others in building your timeline, because you're discussing the case with them in that situation.
- This will be of great assistance to your attorney.
- **Above all:**
  - Do not call the *opposing attorney*.
    - There will be many things wrong with the petition or complaint. It will have facts wrong. It will have names wrong. You may not even have been working when things happened.
    - Do not try to fix this by calling the lawyer. Opposing counsel cannot call you lawfully, but if you call him or her, he or she will be sure to make a record of your call and conversation.
  - Do not call the *plaintiff*.

- You may know the plaintiff. You may believe you are friends. You may not understand why they've sued. *Do not make a phone call.* This could be considered harassment.
- Do not call *people related to or who may know the plaintiff. This makes you look like you have something to hide.*
- Do not call or talk to the *other defendants.*
  - The first thing the plaintiff will ask is if you've discussed the case with other defendants. The implication is you got together to get your stories straight. The only way to avoid this is not to discuss the case with anyone.
- Do not call or talk to the *lawyers of the other defendants.*
- Do not sit down with *codefendants and try to "get the stories straight."*
  - Just because the hospital or a codefendant is against the plaintiff does not make them on the same side as you. They have the goal of escaping liability, and if that means throwing you under the bus, they are happy to do it.
  - Because you are an employee, the employer can compel you to meet with their attorney, but only do so in the presence of your attorney.
- Report to your attorney anyone who says that you should "harmonize your testimony" or "harmonize your version of the facts" with what some other witness remembers or says. This may constitute the crime of perjury or suborning perjury, and your attorney will want to know if this happens.

- You will be served with interrogatories through your attorney.
- Interrogatories are questions that are asked under oath.
- Your attorney will likely object to many of the questions.
- The questions that are not objected to will have to be answered.
- Many of these questions are going to be short answers ("Have you ever been convicted of a felony or misdemeanor?").
- Answer all questions honestly.
- An interrogatory answer has the same force and effect as a statement in court.
- The biggest event in the case is likely to be your deposition.
- You prepare for your deposition *with your attorney*. He or she should role play with you and give you a flavor of what a deposition is like.
- Your attorney will instruct you on how to answer questions.
- Your attorney will tell you to always tell the truth.
- Any lawyer who instructs you to tell anything other than the truth should be reported to the state bar.
- Your deposition is taken to determine what you will say at trial.
- Once the deposition is taken, in most cases the case is over with respect to the witnesses.
- Although the case may drag on for another 18 months and expert witnesses may have their depositions taken, in most cases the only time you testify is in your deposition unless your case is one of the very rare ones that goes to trial.

- If your case goes to trial and you need to testify, you testify according to what you said in your deposition. Tell the truth. If you lose, that's why you have malpractice insurance. Do not destroy your honor and risk spending time in prison by telling anything other than the truth.
- Even if you lose, there are always appeals courts. Your insurer will usually decide if it is necessary to appeal.

Resources

You must have your own malpractice insurance policy. If you do not have such a policy, get one from an insurer. Here are three recommendations:

1. Marsh Proliability Company (https://www.pro liability.com/index.html).
2. Lockton Risk Services (http://www.ahc.lockton-ins.com/pl/apply.html?link=pli).
3. Healthcare Providers Service Organization (http://www.hpso.com/professional-liability-insurance/professions-covered.jsp).

Other resources include:

- *The Respiratory Therapists Legal Answer Book.*
- *Malpractice Depositions: Avoiding the Traps*, by Raymond M. Fish and Melvin E. Ehrhardt (Jan. 1987).
- *Avoiding Medical Malpractice: A Physician's Guide to the Law*, by William T. Choctaw (Apr. 11, 2008).
- *Nursing Practice and the Law: Avoiding Malpractice and Other Legal Risks*, by Mary E. O'Keefe (Sep. 2000).
- *Avoiding Malpractice: 10 Rules, 5 Systems, 20 Cases*, by Carolyn Buppert (June 1, 2002).

Mutual Aid and Protection

▓ Overview

Nearly everyone who works in a job with other people knows that from time to time the boss is simply clueless about what is going on, often right underneath his or her nose. Employees get together, elect someone to carry the ball, and send that person in to talk to the boss on their behalf.

In organizations with a healthy tolerance for dissent and disagreement, the boss may be unhappy, but he or she will usually investigate and, in some cases, take action. In the less tolerant administration, the person elected to make the group's troubles known to management often gets labeled a "rabble-rouser" or a "trouble-maker" and frequently gets the axe.

Because firing an employee who acts for the benefit of others under the doctrine of protected concerted activity is unlawful, employees can usually get their job back, if they know where to go. The National Labor Relations Act protects the right of employees to voice concerns to management for the purpose of mutual aid and protection. An employee who does so and gets terminated has 180 days to make a complaint to the NLRB regional office and request their job back.

Prevention

It is worth saying that you do not want to be the person elected to carry the ball. You take a risk when you do this, and you should almost always let someone else do it, unless you are simply tired of your job or enjoy making trouble.

Legal First Aid

- If you go to management with the concerns of other employees, take something in writing that says you are voicing the concerns of other employees.
- The concerns must have something to do with the terms and conditions of employment to be considered "protected concerted activities."
- Although you do not need to have names or signatures on that piece of paper, some evidence that you are acting for mutual aid and protection is necessary and desirable.
- Make sure you keep a copy, and make sure you give a copy to management.
- Do not be confrontational or insubordinate. You can be fired for being insubordinate and no one can do anything.
- Obey all work rules. If the management can catch you in a work rule violation, you can be terminated. So follow the rules on time and do not leave early.
- If disciplined, ask to know the basis of the discipline. Ask to see the basis in writing. If you are being disciplined for speaking out for others and the employer is foolish enough to put this in writing, it is almost a certainty that you will be reinstated.

- Keep in mind that certain employees (supervisors, salaried personnel) do not qualify for the same protection as line workers.
- If disciplined or terminated, make a complaint quickly to the NLRB.
- You may be asked to fill out an affidavit. You may be asked for the names of witnesses or other employees. Provide them.
- If the NLRB rules in your favor, you are entitled to back pay.

Resources

- *The Developing Labor Law: The Board, the Courts, and the National Labor Relations Act*, by John E. Higgins, Peter A. Janus, Barry J. Kearney, and W. V. "Bernie" Siebert (Nov. 21, 2006).
- *National Labor Relations Act*, by National Labor Relations Board (U.S.) (Apr. 18, 2000).
- *Guide to Basic Law and Procedures Under the National Labor Relations Act*, by United States National Labor Relations Board (June 1990).
- Workplace Rights (available online at http://www.nlrb.gov/Workplace_Rights/employee_rights.aspx).

Whistle-Blower Protections

▉ Overview

The concept of the "whistle-blower" has both positive and negative connotations. All our lives we are taught not to be tattletales, but at the same time we are told that we should not keep secrets that might hurt people. The law recognizes this rather unique approach to truth telling and risk management in a variety of ways, but perhaps the most interesting is in the approach it takes to rewarding people who tattle on those who defraud the government.

This section covers several situations: whistleblowing on fraud, on criminal activity, on violations of Emergency Medical Treatment and Active Labor Act (EMTALA), and on violations of the Sarbanes-Oxley Act and the duty of the CCO.

Prevention

In an ideal world we would always be employed and managed by ethical and conscientious people who always told the truth and never took actions that caused problems. But this is not a perfect world. It is often impossible to know, until after you are enmeshed in an organization, that certain of the apples in the barrel are rotten. By then it may be too late to do anything about them other than blow the whistle.

Legal First Aid

Federal False Claims Act

- If you discover evidence that your employer is cheating the federal government, you can, without violating HIPAA, make a record of those claims that you know to be false.
- You do not have to copy records; you can simply make a list of medical record numbers. You should not withdraw any permanent records from the hospital.
- You should copy only those records that you would normally have access to in the normal course of your job.
- You should not assume that you are empowered as a secret agent to search through computer files or desk drawers.
- Once you have as much evidence as you believe you need, you have two potential ways to share that evidence and seek assistance:
  - Take the evidence to the CCO.
  - Take the evidence to an attorney and file a federal False Claims Act case.
- If you take your case to the attorney and file a case under the False Claims Act, certain things happen:
  - The case is filed under seal.
  - You cannot talk about the case while it is under seal.
  - You cannot discuss the case even with your spouse or close friends.
  - You will be interviewed by the federal government as a witness.
  - You may be required to give testimony under oath.

- You will assist the government in prosecuting its claim.
- It will take from 18 months to 6 years to prosecute the action and receive the reward.
- You may be eligible for 15% to 30% of what the government gets back from the employer, depending on whether the government intervenes or lets your attorney handle the matter.
- It is unlawful for your employer to fire you for blowing the whistle.
- Talk to your attorney to find out the best ways to minimize your risk during the case.
- Most states have state False Claims Acts that also pay rewards when the state is the victim of the fraud.

Public Policy Exception for Reporting Criminal Conduct

Note: Much of the following does not apply in Texas, which takes a very narrow view of this exception.

- In most states, Texas excluded, you have the right to report criminal activity by your employer or coworkers and not risk your job.
- In most states the conduct must be illegal (violate the criminal law) as opposed to unlawful (violate the civil law).
- For example, if the supervisor directed you to lie under oath, that would be illegal, and you could not lawfully do that without violating the criminal law.
- By contrast, rewriting, concealing, or destroying a part of the medical record would be unlawful (violates only the civil law).
- Certain statutes may give you additional rights. For example, the nursing home statute in Missouri mandates that nurses make certain

reports, and when fired for making those reports, nurses got their jobs back even though the conduct was merely unlawful as opposed to illegal.

- Sometimes the law splits hairs in this area. If you have concerns about whether to report criminal activity or unlawful activity, contact an attorney to help you make the decision.

EMTALA

- This federal law provides that persons who disclose noncompliance with the Act (e.g., patient dumping, unlawful transfers) cannot be disciplined or terminated.
- Unfortunately, the Act does not provide a "private right of action" under the law, so courts are split as to whether an employee so discharged can sue.
- The employee may be limited to filing an action with the U.S. Department of Health and Human Services for administrative relief (but no damages).
- For this reason violations of EMTALA should be reported first to the CCO and only to some other agency (U.S. Department Health and Human Services, Office of Inspector General) if the CCO does not take action on the complaint.

Sarbanes-Oxley Whistle-Blower Protections

- Sarbanes-Oxley came along after the Enron debacle and was aimed at restoring public trust in financial institutions and other publicly traded companies. It only applies to companies that sell their stock on the national stock exchanges. A 300-bed community hospital is not covered unless it is a member of a chain of a publicly traded corporation.

- Sarbanes-Oxley's protections for whistle-blowers were predicated on the fact that many of the people in Enron and Worldcom knew about the fraud at the heart of their accounting systems but took no action because they were afraid of being fired. Sarbanes-Oxley has increased the protection provided to whistle-blowers exposing corruption in public companies in three areas:
  - Publicly held companies (those that sell stock) are now required to have a mechanism in place to receive the reports of anonymous whistle-blowers. Section 302 of Sarbanes-Oxloy states, "Each audit committee shall establish procedures for the confidential, anonymous submission by employees of the issuer of concerns regarding questionable accounting or auditing matters." In other words, every publicly traded company must have a mechanism to receive anonymous calls that report fraud and misdeeds.
  - After receiving a report, any investigation conducted must comply with section 806 of the Act, which states that "no publicly traded company, or any officer, employee, contractor, subcontractor, or agent of such company may discharge, demote, suspend, threaten, harass, or in any other manner discriminate against an employee in the terms and conditions of employment because of any lawful act done by the employee."
    - What exactly can be considered a threat? This includes everything from losing your job to being demoted. Any suggested retaliation of any kind is a threat.

- What constitutes harassment? Harassment is meant to cover those situations where an employee is assigned to a room by themselves and given nothing to do in the hopes they will simply quit. Harassment includes those actions designed to make someone want to leave the company.
- How do you know the identity of an anonymous whistle-blower? Usually, the circle of people who know about wrongdoing is small, and those doing the wrong are often able to figure out just who it was that blew the whistle on them.

- Sarbanes-Oxley provisions have made it clear that retaliation against whistle-blowers is wrong. 18 USC § 1513(e) makes retaliation a criminal offense punishable by 10 years in prison.

The CCO

- The CCO is an employee of the hospital who is in a unique position.
- The CCO reports not only to the chief executive officer of the corporation, but also to the chairperson of the board.
- The CCO is the chief ethics officer of the organization and is given authority for making sure that the facility is complying with all state and federal laws.
- CCO personnel are usually either attorneys or persons with risk management training.
- CCO personnel are required by law to follow up on all complaints, no matter how small, that relate to criminal acts or unlawful acts by the corporation.

- For example, a mistake in the hospital's wage index caused by a miscalculation could throw off the hospital's wage index and result in thousands of false claims every year.
- Although the false claims here would not be an intentional act of wrongdoing, they would still result in financial harm to the organization.
- The CCO's job is to find those problems and fix them in the way that costs the organization the least amount of money.
- A CCO may not look the other way. A CCO who is directed by the chief executive officer to look the other way has a duty to make a report to the chairperson of the board. If the chairperson of the board makes the same request, the CCO, to preserve his or her own status as an ethical individual, may have to resign.
- Depending on how capable and ethical the CCO is, he or she can often be an employee's best friend when reporting wrongdoing.
- If the CCO is an attorney, usually the investigation performed by him or her cannot be used against the hospital later but can be used internally to fix problems.
- In those situations not involving the possibility of a financial reward (False Claims Act, State False Claims Act), the CCO should be the first person the clinician should consider involving.
- In situations involving criminal wrongdoing, the CCO should be notified right away.

Resources

- *Whistleblowing: When It Works—And Why*, by Roberta Ann Johnson (Dec. 2002).
- *Whistleblowing: A Guide to Government Reward Programs (How to Collect Millions for Reporting Fraud)*, by Joel Hesch (Oct. 2, 2007).

- *Whistleblowing at Work*, by David B. Lewis (Apr. 15, 2001).
- *The Governance, Risk, and Compliance Handbook: Technology, Finance, Environmental, and International Guidance and Best Practices*, by Anthony Tarantino (Mar. 14, 2008).
- *Building a Career in Compliance and Ethics*, by Joseph E. Murphy (Feb. 28, 2007).
- *Interactive Corporate Compliance: An Alternative to Regulatory Compulsion*, by Jay A. Sigler and Joseph Murphy (June 20, 1988).

Allegations of Assault or Battery

Overview

Fewer things are more important to facilities and administrators than protecting patients from harm. Although it is unlawful for patients to assault care givers, it does happen. Caregivers, however, cannot strike back. Patients may not know or appreciate what they are doing. Caregivers are required not to strike back, even if provoked, because of the doctrine in medicine of doing no harm and because hospitals are strictly liable if their employees assault or batter patients.

An assault is considered the threat of an immediate and unpleasant personal contact or touching. A battery is an unpermitted touching. To swing at someone (even if you miss) is an assault. If you connect with them, it is assault and battery. In most situations, the tort of assault merges with the tort of battery, and a person is liable for the more harmful of the two.

More importantly, if you injure a patient through violence, you may be permanently disqualified from working with patients and placed on the Employee Disqualification List in your state. Such a disqualification can result in the loss of your license.

Prevention

Manage your emotions and your temper at work. If you get frustrated, walk away, cool down, talk to a colleague, or call your spouse. Under no circumstances should you hit a patient, a family member, or a guest or visitor, no matter how much they may deserve it.

If you are assaulted at work by a patient or family member:

- Do not resist.
- Cover your head and face with your hands and withdraw as quickly as possible.
- Yell for help from coworkers.
- Ask security to come to your assistance.
- Do not hit back.
- Do not attempt to block blows because this may be interpreted as a physical assault.
- If another coworker is assaulted in front of you, use nonviolent means to break up the assault.
- Do not attempt to intercede between two people who are fighting.
- Contact law enforcement as soon as possible.
- If a visitor or family member instigated the assault, have that visitor or family member escorted off the premises by the police and barred from the facility by security.
- Seek medical attention if required.
- Make a full report.
- If injured, have employee health make a full report.
- Cooperate with law enforcement if required.
- Complete Appendix 1 for your records.

Legal First Aid

Sometimes reactions are reflexive and not the product of true intention. When we touch a hot stove, we draw back. When someone tries to punch us, we duck and throw up an arm. All of these responses are preprogrammed and never thought about. But, in the context of an assault claim, these reactions may become serious issues. If you make contact with a patient either out of anger or accident, do the following:

- Contact an attorney immediately. Give him or her the facts. Let him or her guide you.
- Go over the facts with your attorney before making any entries in the medical record or filling out any paperwork.
- Report any injury to the patient to appropriate personnel.
- Do not involve yourself in the patient's care from that point forward.
- Do not give a statement to anyone without your attorney present.
- An allegation that you assaulted or battered a patient is a serious allegation that, if proved, will likely end your career. The best first aid is a good lawyer, and getting his or her advice quickly can be career saving.

Resources

- *Respiratory Therapists Legal Answer Book.*
- *Humane Pressure Point Self-Defense: Dillman Method for Law Enforcement, Medical Personnel, Business Professionals, Men and Women,* by George A. Dillman (Aug. 17, 2001).

Slander and Libel

■ Overview

Slander is a spoken untruth told for the purposes of harming an individual. Libel is the publication of an untruthful statement about someone, again, with the purpose of causing them harm. Health care workers can be liable for either the tort of slander or the tort of libel if they knowingly engage in telling falsehoods about patients, visitors, vendors, coworkers, or others.

Although the law makes a showing of holding people accountable for untruthful statements, there are more holes in the law of libel and slander than there are in your average serving of Swiss cheese. Whereas people often threaten one another with libel and slander lawsuits, the fact is very few ever get brought because these lawsuits frequently do not have any real chance of success.

Prevention

Writing in a patient record a statement about a patient you know to be untrue can be libel, just the way that speaking that statement to another coworker can be slander. For this reason the best way to prevent these kinds of situations is to be rigorous in applying the truth test to what we speak and write about patients in the hospital.

Also, a statement of fact is actionable. If a person says, "Dr. Jones is a murderer," that statement is phrased as a statement of fact, and if Dr. Jones is not a murderer, then he could potentially sue for slander (or libel if written). However, "In my opinion, because Dr. Jones does abortions, he is a murderer," is a statement of opinion that is protected by the First Amendment of the Constitution. Most people cannot distinguish between those two statements, and as a result it is just never a good idea to go around making statements of that nature.

Truth is a complete defense to libel or slander. Thus if Dr. Jones truly is a murderer and this can be proved, then there is a good defense to the charge of libel. However, because it costs a lot of money to defend any lawsuit, it is a very good idea not to rely on truth as the ultimate defense when discretion is the better part of valor in every situation.

Legal First Aid

- If someone threatens to sue you over a slanderous or libelous statement, consult a lawyer immediately.
- Provide the attorney with all the facts.
- With the attorney, examine the statement.
- If the statement is objectively true, do not be alarmed.
- If the statement is written and is not objectively true, you should do your best to retract the statement if your lawyer so advises.
- If you do receive a summons or complaint about the statement, take it to your attorney to handle.
- In addition to the defense of truth, there are numerous other defenses:

- Privilege (you had a right or obligation to make the statement which you believed to be true in order to protect another person).
- Publication by accident (you did not intend to publish the statement to others).
- Consent to the publication (the person complaining gave permission to have the information published).
- Lack of damages (the person claiming libel was not injured by the statement).
- Some people who are notorious (like Osama bin Laden or Theodore Kaczynski) are considered to be "libel proof," meaning that there is no lie that could be told that would injure their reputation any more than the truth already has.

- In most cases if you are sued over libel or slander and the conduct does not relate to your workplace activities, you may have coverage under your homeowners' policy of insurance.

Resources

- *Insult to Injury: Libel, Slander, and Invasions of Privacy*, by William K. Jones (Nov. 2003).
- *The Law of Defamation and the Internet*, by Matthew Collins (Feb. 2, 2006).

Unlawful Restraint

■ Overview

No person may be held against his or her will or confined under our system of justice without due process of law. This right, enshrined in both the Fifth and Fourteenth Amendments to the Constitution of the United States, makes it wrong for someone to take away our liberty without just cause. Just as the police cannot restrain an individual without just cause, a facility cannot restrain an individual without just cause, even if doing so may ultimately be in his or her best interests.

Sometimes hospitals and hospital employees think of their roles as patient protectors in ways that put them at odds with this concept. The patient who wants to smoke when it is 15 degrees outside and who refuses to come back inside may be violating hospital rules and engaging in conduct sure to make his health condition worse. But he cannot be forcibly restrained and brought back in the facility. Similarly, the 90-year-old who from time to time does inappropriate things with his hands cannot be restrained without a proper medical diagnosis and only after following the rules regarding the imposition of restraints.

Prevention

Restraints should never be used unless necessary, and the only time they are necessary is when their use is a necessary adjunct to the treatment of the disease or condition for which that patient is being treated. In other words, patients cannot be restrained because it is more convenient for the staff or because the family wants them restrained. They can only be restrained in the least restrictive environment, and only for a length of time that is reasonable under hospital policies and protocols as guided by state and federal law.

The decision to use restraints must be balanced against the medical need and the likelihood that the patient will harm him- or herself or others. Once the decision is made, it must be revisited at regular intervals until the restraints can be removed.

A patient who wishes to leave a hospital or a room or a facility must be allowed to do so unless he or she has been adjudged incompetent. Although an Alzheimer's victim can be confined to a locked unit because of their medical condition, a person without such a disease could not be locked in a unit simply because it was more convenient for the staff or for the patient's family.

Legal First Aid

- If you are required to use restraints, document the need.
- Your documentation should explain why the restraint is needed.
- Your documentation should explain what intermediate steps were taken before resorting to restraints.
- Your documentation should lay out why the restraints used are the least restrictive environment that can be used for the patient.

- Make sure you have a physician's order.
- Make sure you and the physician revisit that order as required by state and federal law, usually every 72 hours.
- If a complaint is lodged about restraint use by a family member or relative, make sure that you document the complaint, fill out an incident report, and complete Appendix 1 for your own use.
- If a federal or state investigator comes to investigate, make sure you consult with your attorney before answering any questions.

Resources
- *The Respiratory Therapist's Legal Answer Book.*
- American Geriatrics Society: Position Statement on Restraint Use (available online at http://www.americangeriatrics.org/products/positionpapers/restraintsupdate.shtml).

Health Care Contracts

■ Overview

Contracts are really nothing more than promises. The difference between the contract and the promise is simply that a contract is a promise that a court will enforce. So much is written about contracts and so little is understood.

What you need to know about a contract—any contract—is that when you enter into one you are making a promise that you may later be hauled in to court about. Contracts can be verbal or written. Written contracts are easier for courts to enforce, and certain contracts cannot lawfully be made verbally (e.g., contracts for the sale of land).

The most important thing to know about contracts in the health care context, instead of the personal context, is that when you make a contract with another entity, depending on your status in the organization, you may be binding the organization. That is why most contracting is done only through a designated person in the Supply or Material Management Section.

Prevention

The best way to prevent contract woes is simply to read everything you sign that purports to be a contract. Ask questions about what the contract says and what it means. If the salesperson says that something written into the contract only applies in certain instances but the contract does not state that, the words of the salesperson will not hold up in court. Read everything. Understand everything.

Also keep in mind that with regard to contracts between commercial entities, there is a wide body of law under what is called the Uniform Commercial Code. The Uniform Commercial Code has been adopted in nearly every state in the country (Louisiana being the only notable exception). It governs contracts, and it has some provisions that are somewhat counterintuitive. If you are buying a piece of equipment and do not understand the disclaimer of warranties in the sales contract, it is a good idea to get a legal opinion on this issue.

In most cases the only way to truly understand everything a contract involves is to get a legal opinion from a lawyer about whether to enter into a contract or not. Most misunderstandings, disputes, and legal cases could have been avoided if the parties had either understood what the contract said or understood what the contract meant in the first place.

Legal First Aid

Presented With a Contract

- If someone presents you with a contract, your first step is to read it carefully.
- Understand what it says.
- If it says something you don't agree with, line that sentence or paragraph out and initial it. If the other side wants it in, they can refuse to do the deal. If they don't object, your modification becomes part of the contract.
- If you have questions about the contract and someone says that a provision only applies to a

certain situation, get that explanation in writing. An explanation not in writing does you no good in court if you have to enforce the contract later.

- If you need to modify the contract in some way, don't modify it with a handshake. Most contracts have provisions that make any verbal modification void.
- Before you sign a contract, unless there is no alternative, get your family lawyer to review the document and explain it to you.

Someone Claims You Breached a Contract

- If someone claims you breached a contract and there is no lawsuit, then:
  - Have them explain what they believe is the breach.
  - If possible, "cure" the breach. For example, in an installment loan contract you can breach the agreement by not paying a payment on time. You can cure that breach by paying the missed payment.
- If the breach cannot be cured, you should seek legal counsel.
- Seek out an attorney with expertise in contract law and litigation.

You Believe Someone Breached a Contract

- Read the contract. Then reread the contract.
- You must follow the terms of the contract explicitly.
- The rights and remedies are likely spelled out in the contract.
- You may have an obligation to give notice to the other side of the breach in order to sue or recover.

- You may have to give the other side an opportunity to cure its breach.
- If you cannot get the other side to cure its breach, your only recourse may be to sue.
- Contact an attorney who handles breach of contract litigation and get his or her help and opinion.

You Need to Have a Contract Drafted

- Do not get a form contract from the Internet or from a legal form book.
- Go to an attorney and have an attorney draft the contract for you.
- It may cost more to use an attorney, but a form book will not defend you in court if the other side breaches the agreement.
- If you draft your own contract, remember that the person who represents him- or herself has a fool for a client.

Resources

- *Understanding Contracts* (Understanding Series [New York]), by Jeffrey Thomas Ferriell and Michael J. Navin (June 2004).
- *Contracts: Examples and Explanations* (Examples and Explanations Series), by Brian A. Blum (Mar. 2004).
- *Contracts*, by John D. Calamari and Joseph M. Perillo (June 2004).
- *Contracts in a Nutshell*, by Anthony M. Skrocki (May 30, 2006).
- *Understanding Contracts for Dummies*, Wiley Publishing (2008).

Covenants Not to Compete

■ Overview

The contract that provides that an individual must compete is a specific kind of contract with some specific kinds of issues and requires some specific guidance. Generally, it is never in an employee's interest to sign a covenant not to compete. Covenants work fine to protect the employer, but they make it nearly impossible for a professional to seek employment in the area covered by the agreement. Although such agreements are required to be reasonable in time and geographical scope, some courts have enforced agreements that are much broader than reasonable.

In most cases a covenant is sought where the employee has access to sensitive information or data that the employer considers "proprietary." Things like patient lists, treatment protocols, physician coverage schedules, and similar data may all be considered "trade secrets" if not well known in the community. An employer wants to protect itself in the event it has to fire a popular employee (like a manager) who might then be hired across town and take away large numbers of the hospital's staff. In this situation, they will ask for a covenant not to compete.

Like anything else, when someone wants something, they must be willing to pay for it. If a covenant is not discussed during the interview and is not brought up until after the employee reports for work, in some cases it may not be valid. If the employer wants it, he or she has to pay some consideration—usually money—to obtain it.

I routinely advise clients not to sign these agreements. In most cases, that is the proper legal advice. However, if people want the job that is being offered, they have no choice but to sign the document. The advice that follows is predicated on this simple fact: In most cases if you want the job you have to agree to the terms. If you agree to the terms when you're hired, even though they're unfair, you cannot later say you didn't agree or understand the documents.

Prevention

The best way to avoid problems with a contract that requires you not to compete as a price of getting a job is to walk away. In some cases you may believe that the offer of salary and benefits is substantial enough to justify the risk. In nearly all cases you will be mistaken. When an employer asks for a covenant not to compete, in almost all instances the interests it is protecting is the interest in controlling employee behavior. This is because a covenant not to compete applies regardless of whether you quit your job or are fired. So although a covenant may be aimed at stopping Hospital A from nabbing the lab manager from Hospital B, it also prevents Hospital A from hiring that manager if he or she steps on an administrator's toes and gets fired.

If you have to sign a covenant not to compete, it should be the narrowest possible agreement, and it should be negotiated by an attorney so that there is a record of what was discussed and how the agreement came together.

Legal First Aid

Presented With a Contract Not to Compete

- If someone presents you with a contract not to compete, your first step is to read it carefully. Then read it again. It is vital that you understand what it says as well as what it does not say:
    - Does the contract or covenant apply only to a reasonable geographical area?
        - For example, "Employee may not compete with Company X in the St. Louis metropolitan area."
    - Or does it provide a larger geographical area that might make it hard for you to find new work if you were let go? Can you live with it?
    - Determine if the contract is for a reasonable time.
        - For example, "Employee agrees not to compete for a period of 1 year."
    - Or is it more imposing? Can you live with it if things go badly?
        - For example, "Employee is forbidden from working as a laboratory manager for a period of 10 years commencing on the date of termination."
    - Determine if the contract is negotiable. Can you alter the terms in any way?
    - Determine what happens if you are terminated for other than cause.
        - Does the contract provide for severance so as to permit you not to work for the time specified?
    - What are the stated bases for the noncompetition (e.g., trade secrets)?

- Does the contract provide for a different result if the company downsizes or termi-
  nates employment for other than just cause
  (e.g., layoffs)?
- If you are unwilling to move out of the geographical area at the end of employment, do not
  sign the contract. If you wind up terminated,
  you will have to move.
- Have your attorney review any contract and
  evaluate it in terms of the state law where the
  contract is made.
- Be aware that you may be "enjoined" by a court
  and legally required not to work in your chosen
  field.
- Keep in mind that in some contracts there are
  "liquidated damages" clauses that impose a
  penalty of $100 or more per day for violations.

Someone Claims You Breached a Contract Not to Compete

- If someone claims you breached a contract not
  to compete and there is no lawsuit, then:
  - Have them explain what they believe is the
    breach.
  - If possible, "cure" the breach, for example,
    by changing jobs.
  - If the breach cannot be cured, you should
    seek legal counsel.
  - You should seek out someone with expertise
    in employment law and litigation.

Resources

- *Covenants Not to Compete*, 5th Edition (2007
  Supplement), by Brian M. Malsberger (Nov. 9,
  2007).

- *Covenants Not to Compete: A State-by-State Survey*, by American Bar Association. Employment Rights and Responsibilities Committee, Brian M. Malsberger, Samuel M. Brock, and Arnold H. Pedowitz (Nov. 2002).
- *Understanding Contracts* (Understanding Series [New York]), by Jeffrey Thomas Ferriell and Michael J. Navin (June 2004).
- *Covenants Not to Compete*, by Mark R. Filipp (Sep. 22, 2005).
- *Contracts: Examples and Explanations* (Examples and Explanations Series), by Brian A. Blum (Mar. 2004).
- *Covenants Not to Compete* (Volumes 1 and 2), by Kurt Decker (1998).
- *Contracts*, by John D. Calamari and Joseph M. Perillo (June 2004).
- *Contracts in a Nutshell*, by Anthony M. Skrocki (May 30, 2006).
- *Covenants Not to Compete* (Employment Law Library), by Anthony C. Valiulis (Jan. 15, 1986).
- *Understanding Contracts for Dummies*, Wiley Publishing (2008).

Consumer Fraud

Overview

In most states the "Little FTC Act" or Merchandising Practices Statute makes advertisements or statements intended for marketing subject to strict standards of honesty, good faith, and fair dealing. If the statements made in marketing materials are false, deceptive, or create false promises, they may be actionable under these powerful consumer fraud statutes. Missouri's Merchandising Practices Act, for example, states as follows:

> 407.020. 1. The act, use or employment by any person of any deception, fraud, false pretense, false promise, misrepresentation, unfair practice or the concealment, suppression, or omission of any material fact in connection with the sale or advertisement of any merchandise in trade or commerce . . . is declared to be an unlawful practice. . . . Any act, use or employment declared unlawful by this subsection violates this subsection whether committed before, during or after the sale, advertisement or solicitation.

The statute does not define the terms fraud, false pretense, false promise, misrepresentation, or unfair practice. Instead, regulations promulgated by the Attorney General define those terms, and they define them very broadly. Deception is defined as "any method, act, use, practice, advertisement or solicitation that has the tendency or capacity to mislead, deceive or cheat, or that tends to create a false impression." The regulations go on to say that neither reliance nor an intent to mislead or deceive are necessary elements of deception. Therefore any statement with the capacity to mislead or deceive, whether it is intended to deceive or not, is considered to violate the state law with regard to deceptive practices.

The regulations in Missouri define an unfair practice as any practice that either "offends public policy" (derived from state statute or the Federal Trade Commission) or is "unethical, oppressive or unscrupulous" and presents a risk of harm to consumers. The regulations go on to state that a person does not need to prove deception or fraud to prove unfair practices. Thus the use of arbitration agreements that tie admission to signing the arbitration agreement, or other acts that deprive a resident of free choice, often violate the state's merchandising statutes.

The law attempts to regulate consumer transactions. It is aimed at restoring some balance between big businesses and the individual consumer. However, the law uses a rather odd twist. If a statement is true when made (for example, the statement "we protect patients from falls") and the statement later proves false (a patient suffers a fall), the fact that the statement was true when it was made is no defense because the statute is violated "whether [the act is] committed before, during or after the sale, advertisement or solicitation."

Prevention

The best way to prevent consumer fraud allegations is to be honest in dealing with the public and not to make statements that might be misconstrued. If a

- Get legal advice about whether you need to show up, and if you do, make a point of going in the best clothes you have, just as if you were going to church. The court is to be addressed as "your honor" and anyone else is a "sir" or a "ma'am."
- Usually, if you ask for additional time to get a lawyer, the court will let you do that.
- Don't go it alone. Get legal help if needed.

Resources

- *Respiratory Therapists Legal Answer Book*, by Anthony L. DeWitt (2005).

Overview

Small claims courts were an innovation in the 1970s that permitted average citizens to take small matters before judges who would decide the law on the basis of the facts as told by the parties, without a whole lot of evidentiary objection and courtroom shenanigans. It is a system that works very well, whether you are on the plaintiff's or defendant's end of things. In most cases the case is limited to a certain value (in Missouri $3,000, some other states as much as $10,000). This keeps the damage inflicted from being excessive (in most cases) if you lose but gives a fair sense of justice if you win.

Prevention

Deal with people fairly, treat them well, and verify the bona fides of people you do business with before you do business and you may never need a small claims court. But if you are the victim of a scam or a fraud, you have the ability to go to court on your own if the value is less than the jurisdictional amount.

Legal First Aid

- The following applies regardless of whether you are a plaintiff or a defendant in small claims court:
  - Do your homework.

- If you are sued or are going to sue someone in small claims court, call the courthouse and find out when this court is conducted.
- Then go and watch.
- Watch how people present their cases and what works and what doesn't work.
- Do the research.
  - Both Lexis and Westlaw (http://www.westlaw.com) allow people with a credit card to use their legal research network.
  - Both have "natural language" searches that permit you to search the law in a given state for cases that deal with a particular topic.
  - Searches like "can a landlord retain a tenant's deposit" will often yield lots of cases that may help (or may hurt) your case.
  - Doing this before you go to court can help you avoid a bad outcome.
  - Follow the forms. Use the forms provided by the court to file your lawsuit.
- Write your complaint in numbered paragraphs. Provide the following information in the following order without embellishment (no angry words):
  - Who you are
  - Who the other side is
  - When the events at issue began
  - What the other side did to you
  - Why what they did is wrong
  - Explain how much money you have lost
  - Ask the court for judgment

- Pay the filing fee and have the sheriff serve the other side. You usually have to pay a fee for this service too.
- If the other side is a business, you need to find out if they are incorporated or if they are a sole proprietorship.
- You do this through the state. In most cases the secretary of state has a list of all the corporations and their "registered agents."
- This registered agent is the person who must be served.
- If the registered agent is in another city, you have to get the sheriff in that county to serve the complaint.
- You will get a court date. Show up on that date. Often, the case will not be heard on that day if the other side objects.
- When the day arrives, stand up and tell the judge what happened. Answer his or her questions. Sit down when told. Do not argue when the other side is talking. Let them have their time. Politely ask for a chance to respond when they are finished.
- If you are defending, you do not have to file an answer in most cases.
- Show up and tell your side of the story.
- Again, no angry words. Speak plainly and calmly, even if the other side calls you names and says bad things about you. Remember that everything you say must be the truth.
- If the judgment is for you, you can get help from the clerk in collecting it.
- If the judgment is against you, you can usually appeal. Each court has different rules about appeals.

Resources

- *Everybody's Guide to Small Claims Court,* by Ralph E. Warner (Mar. 30, 2008).
- *Represent Yourself in Court: How to Prepare and Try a Winning Case,* by Paul Bergman, Sara J. Berman-Barrett, and Lisa Guerin (Jan. 31, 2006).
- *Small Claims Court Guidebook* (Entrepreneur Legal Guides), by Michael Spadaccini (Nov. 21, 2007).
- *Winning in Small Claims Courts: A Step-By-Step Guide for Trying Your Own Small Claims Cases,* by William E. Brewer (Nov. 1998).

Breach of Contract

Overview

In the context of personal affairs, contracts are a normal part of everyday life. When we finance a car or home, we enter a contract. When we buy insurance, we buy a contract that gives us rights. Sometimes even when we enter employment, we get a contract. Even when you drop your car off for an oil change, even though nothing is written, you are entering into a contract where you promise to pay them for changing the oil and they promise to change your oil in a competent manner. Contracts are everywhere, whether you know it or not.

Prevention

As with contracts in the employment context and dealing with issues in health care, it is important for all parties to read a contract before signing it. If you have never read your insurance contract on your house or car, do it today. You will be amazed at the things that are not covered.

Legal First Aid

Signing the Contract

- Contracts must be read and understood.
- Do your homework before you sign.

- If you sign a contract, you're agreeing to its terms and that includes all its terms, even if you don't know it.
- If a contract form is printed, always check the back.
- Never agree to a contract with an arbitration clause ("I promise to arbitrate any disputes with XYZ Company arising out of this contract . . . ") unless you know and understand that you're giving up your right to go to court.
- Understand that most commercial contracts require you to pay the attorney's fees if you breach the contract.
- Understand your rights.
- Some language in contracts is simply too technical to be understood by the layperson. This is why there are lawyers.
- If you do not understand what a contract means, get a legal opinion.
- If you're signing a contract to buy a car, for example, know what you are buying, who has what obligations at what times, and what the remedies of each side are in the event one of you backs out.
- Doing this before you sign can help you avoid a bad outcome.

Form Contracts

- Most contracts are form contracts; no one selling you anything expects or wants you to read them.
- Frankly, it may be a waste of your time to read an installment loan contract because they all say pretty much the same thing: you are borrowing money, this is what it's going to cost you, and this is what will happen if you don't pay it back.

- But you should read the contract anyway because at some point you may have an issue with the loan and need to know what your rights are.
- Things to look for in written contracts:
  - Does the contract apportion the risk of loss?
    - If the risk of loss passes to you on signing the contract (for example, when buying a car or a house), then the need to insure the property arises at the time of signing.
  - Does the contract provide for liquidated damages?
    - Some contracts specify a penalty or liquidated damages for certain conduct (e.g., late payment).
    - Understanding the grace periods provided in such contracts is very important. Does the contract provide a window of opportunity to unwind the contract?
    - Some consumer contracts are required to provide grace periods (usually 72 hours) for you to "undo" a deal. If this is the case, it will be in the contract. If not, it won't be. Don't assume you have a time to undo the contract if that is not spelled out in the document. Does the contract provide for where to give notice?
    - Some contracts provide for ways to give notice and for instances in which notice must be given.
    - A lease may require you to give 2 months notice before renewing it.
    - A cell phone contract may provide that it can be canceled at any time but that notice must be given to a particular

person. Does the contract provide an indemnity agreement?

- Some contracts, especially leases, contain indemnity agreements which provide that you will indemnify the owner if someone sues the owner because of what you do.

- If you have such an agreement, you should have insurance to protect you against this possibility. Does the contract disclaim warranties?

- Some sellers' contracts disclaim warranties. For example, a lease contract might well disclaim that the car you are leasing is fit for a particular purpose (like, let's say, driving). If you lease the car and the car is not useful for this purpose, a disclaimer of warranties may make it impossible for you to get the problem remedied. Does the contract provide for specific remedies?

- Some contracts provide that on breach certain specific remedies apply.

- Know and understand what those remedies are. Does the contract impair your legal remedies?

- In most situations where you are buying a device or product, if you are injured you can sue the seller and the manufacturer.

- Certain contracts may limit your rights to sue.

- Arbitration agreements are very common in this context.

- If you find yourself in a situation where you have to breach an installment loan contract:

- Go to the lender first and tell them what the problem is.
- Most lenders will work with you.
- Be up front and renegotiate the terms of the loan; avoid default if at all possible.
- If you overextend:
  - Seek help from consumer credit services that will restructure your debts.
  - Seek bankruptcy protection if at all possible.
- If someone fails to honor a contract you made with them:
  - See an attorney.
  - If the matter is small, you may want to go to small claims court.
  - The money you spend and the time you spend on the front end of reading and understanding (and getting a legal opinion on) any contract will be time and money well spent if there is a problem later.

Resources

- *What Do You Mean It's Not Covered?: A Practical Guide to Understanding Insurance in a High Risk World*, 1st edition, by James Walsh (May 1995).
- *Understanding, Creating, and Implementing Contracts*, by Laurel A. Vietzen (Aug. 2007).
- *Understanding Sales, Leases, and Licenses in a Global Perspective*, by Michael L. Rustad (Nov. 6, 2007).

Debtor–Creditor Relationships

▇ Overview

Of all the legal predicaments that threaten to ruin your life and destroy your peace of mind, getting into debt without a way to get out is the worst. Debt problems spill over into marital problems. Those spill over into employment problems. The loss of a job makes it hard to continue to make payments, which accelerates the problems. If you don't have money problems currently, read the Prevention part of this section. If you already have money problems, read the First Aid section.

Prevention

When Ben Franklin suggested we should be neither a lender nor a borrower he was giving good advice. To the extent possible, I never finance anything unless I simply cannot afford it or unless someone else is making the payments. This requires a habit of saving, and the discipline to buy only those things that you need to buy to live a happy and healthy life. If I had a dollar for every stupid thing I have purchased since age 18, I would never need to play the lottery.

The best way to prevent problems with creditors is to have none or to keep the list of them so small that you can manage what you have. I have a house loan and two credit cards that I use. One is for business, the other for personal use. The personal use card is used only for convenience purposes. It is easier to charge a wedding dress than wait the 30 minutes for someone to call in a $1,300 check for a wedding dress. When the bill comes in, I pay it off immediately. As a result, I rarely incur charges for interest. I make the same habit in my business card, settling up expenses at the end of the month when I get an expense check from my employer.

No one starts out thinking they will get in debt. It doesn't happen with one purchase, it happens on the hundredth unthinking purchase. Use credit cards for convenience, not as a source of financing.

Acquiring the habit of saving is a hard thing to do. But you have to put back money every week for those times when something unforeseen happens. You have an accident. A drive shaft goes out. Your son or daughter needs college tuition. This is not difficult to do, but it does require discipline.

The fewer creditors you have, the fewer people you have to worry about paying. This is what leads to peace of mind. If you do not know how to set up a budget and discipline your spending, there are numerous resources available online and in the public domain. See Resources on page 191.

Legal First Aid

Dire Straights

- You are using your Mastercard to pay Visa and your Visa to pay Discover. What on earth can you do? Here are the best recommendations:
  - Go to Consumer Credit Counseling Service. This is a nonprofit agency that can and will help you.

- Do not go to a private ("for profit") credit counseling service. Often, these services are no more than debt consolidation loan companies who want to sell you more debt.
- If you cannot find an agency locally, beware of those that are online. Many are no more than scam artists who will steal your credit card information and exacerbate your problems.
- If your liabilities (the amount of money you owe) are greater than your assets (the amount of money you can reasonably pay and still put diapers on the kids), then your best solution may be bankruptcy.
- With the reform of bankruptcy laws, however, you now have to first start by trying to consolidate your debt or restructure it through a counseling service.
- If you believe bankruptcy is the only option for you, see an attorney who handles these and, in most cases, one who handles only these kinds of cases.
- I'm just a month or 2 behind, what do I do?
  - If you are struggling and are behind but not so bad that you cannot catch up, then the best thing you can do is to get help from a counseling service.
  - Even if you don't use their credit counseling, you still might find their budget advice helpful.
  - Also keep in mind that it may be necessary to secure a second job or work longer hours. If you can do this and pay off your balances, you may be able to learn a very important lesson.
- Collection agencies are after me!

- If you have started to receive calls, particularly calls at work, you need credit counseling help. Do that before doing any of the following:
  - When you receive a call about a debt, find out first if the caller is part of the creditor's office (the Mastercard people, for example) or an outside collection agency (Acme Collections).
  - If the creditor is calling, be honest, ask for help, and try to work through the problem.
  - If the collection agency is calling, expect the collector to:
    - Attempt to bully you.
    - Tell you that all kinds of bad things are going to happen.
    - Demand you pay an amount Donald Trump couldn't afford.
    - Threaten to call your boss.
  - All of these things, however, are unlawful.
  - A collector is required by 15 USC § 1692 to treat you with respect and never to be unprofessional or unkind to you.
  - You have a right not to be contacted at work if you have some other means of being contacted. If the collector calls at work, you should:
    - Tell the collector not to call at work.
    - Get the fax number of the collector and fax them a letter telling them not to call you at work.
    - Send the letter by fax and by certified mail.

- If you continue to receive calls at work after the letter, consult an attorney.
- You have a right not to be contacted at all. See the sample letter to a collector (Appendix 4).

- You should know that the Fair Debt Collection Practices Act requires that debt collectors treat you fairly and prohibits certain methods of debt collection. Of course, the law does not erase any legitimate debt you owe.
- Collectors cannot:
  - Use threats of violence or harm.
  - Publish a list of consumers who refuse to pay their debts (except to a credit bureau).
  - Use obscene or profane language.
  - Repeatedly use the telephone to annoy someone.
- Debt collectors may not use any false or misleading statements when collecting a debt. For example, debt collectors may not:
  - Falsely imply that they are attorneys or government representatives.
  - Falsely imply that you have committed a crime.
  - Falsely represent that they operate or work for a credit bureau.
  - Misrepresent the amount of your debt.
  - Indicate that papers being sent to you are legal forms when they are not.
  - Indicate that papers being sent to you are not legal forms when they are.
- Debt collectors also may not state that:

- You will be arrested if you do not pay your debt.
- They will seize, garnish, attach, or sell your property or wages, unless the collection agency or creditor intends to do so, and it is legal to do so.
- Actions, such as a lawsuit, will be taken against you, when such action legally may not be taken, or when they do not intend to take such action.
- Debt collectors may not:
    - Give false credit information about you to anyone, including a credit bureau.
    - Send you anything that looks like an official document from a court or government agency when it is not.
    - Use a false name.
- Debt collectors may not engage in unfair practices when they try to collect a debt. For example, collectors may not:
    - Collect any amount greater than your debt, unless your state law permits such a charge.
    - Deposit a post-dated check prematurely.
    - Use deception to make you accept collect calls or pay for telegrams.
    - Take or threaten to take your property unless this can be done legally.
    - Contact you by postcard.
- You have a right to contact the Federal Trade Commission (http://www.ftc.gov) if you have been treated improperly by a collection agent. Keep in mind that you may also have a right to sue such a collector. The amount of the penalty (up to $1,000

per violation) may exceed the amount of the debt they are attempting to collect.

Resources

- Appendix 4: Letter to Collector.
- *Fair Debt Collection Practices: Federal and State Law and Regulation*, by Manuel H. Newburger and Barbara Barron (June 2002).
- *Fair Debt Collection* (The Consumer Credit and Sales Legal Practice Series), by Robert J. Hobbs, O. Randolph Bragg, and National Consumer Law Center.
- Consumer Credit Counseling Services (available online at http://www.cccsatl.org).

Domestic Relations Law

▨ Overview

Of all the trials that face modern couples today, the one that presents the greatest challenge is maintaining a happy and productive marriage. According to the most recent statistics nearly 2.3 million people got married in 2005, whereas that same year 3.6 people per thousand got divorced. As of 2003 44% of custodial mothers and 56% of custodial fathers were separated or divorced, and 7.8 million Americans paid approximately $40 billion in child support payments. Of the persons making support payments, 84% were male. Only about 20% of couples reach their 35th wedding anniversary. About five and a half million people live together without benefit of marriage.

In most court systems divorce and child custody cases make up nearly 40% of the cases filed in the courts every year. Thirty percent of cases involving child support involve more than one state's law.

There is no easy way to go through a divorce. Although it may provide a well of inspiration for country singers, divorce is a tough and brutal process that involves unwinding a relationship that is both personal and financial. Whereas two can live as cheaply as one, they cannot do it after a divorce. Nearly everyone who goes through a divorce suffers credit problems and has difficulties in either making or receiving child support payments.

As is often true in these matters, what you do in the first 4 hours after you decide to obtain a divorce is often the key to whether you have a good experience or a bad experience

Prevention

If I had a dollar for every person who told me their lawyer messed up their divorce, I would not need to write books. Lawyers are frequently blamed for screwing things up, and frankly, they are all too often to blame. But in most of the cases I have seen, it is the failure to take the lawyer's advice that ultimately determines whether you come out of a divorce with something more than the clothes on your back.

Getting a divorce is a tough and momentous decision. Once made, it can rarely be retracted. Lives of both the participants (husbands and wives) as well as the noncombatants (children and in-laws) are forever affected. The time to apply thought to the issue of divorce is in the days and weeks before you make the decision. Once the decision is made, you should approach it as irrevocable. There is good reason for this. First, the person you are seeking a divorce from knows every button to push on you and may have made a lifelong habit of manipulating you. They may manipulate you further if you do not make the decision irrevocable. Second, if you delay, reconsider, delay some more, and wait to pull the trigger, you may find yourself in an unfriendly forum, without resources to defend yourself, and the victim of a legal mugging.

The best way to prevent self-injury in domestic relations matters is to be sure this is what you want at the beginning and then take definitive and irrevocable action to implement the plan. And although not all rattlesnakes rattle before the strike, those that do often get shot. Learn from the snakes. Do not threaten, discuss, or ponder out loud the concept of divorce. Instead, get legal advice and let your lawyer announce your plans after you have taken measures to safeguard your income, property, and possessions.

People who are threatened with divorce sometimes do strange things. In short, rational people with a history of acting rationally tend to act completely irrationally when the most significant relationship in their life goes south.

It is for this reason, as harsh and cruel as it sounds, that you have to protect yourself first and not extend the courtesy that you would normally extend to someone you have cared deeply about.

Legal First Aid
The single most important thing you can do in getting a divorce is find the best domestic relations lawyer and have that lawyer represent you.

Finding a Lawyer
- Talk to people who have recently been divorced about their experiences with their lawyers. Find out who they used.
- Get referrals from people in the legal community. Your lawyer's divorce lawyer will be one of the best in town.
- Talk frankly and up front about fees and retainers.
- A lawyer will usually want a retainer to cover costs for the first 6 months of the case. Some divorces can be handled in weeks, others take years. Be prepared to pay handsomely for good representation.

- If you are the nonearning spouse, you may be able to afford good representation if your spouse makes a good income. Sometimes attorneys will work for less money up front with the idea that one spouse (the one with more assets) will pay the attorney's fees of the other. In some states this is a matter of statute, whereas in others it is up to the judge. Usually, it is part of any settlement.
- You want a lawyer who knows the law and who knows the judge involved in the case.
- There are plenty of lawyers willing to promise to fight to the death on every little thing.
- Why wouldn't they? Every time they file a pleading or make a phone call on your behalf they are charging you at rates around $250 per hour.
- If you want to fight over everything, it makes them money.
- You want a lawyer who is a good communicator and negotiator, not someone who wants to put notches on their gunbelt.
- All a lawyer like that will do is run up a huge bill, and when you cannot pay it, he or she will withdraw, leaving you at the mercy of your soon-to be-ex-spouse's lawyer. Not a good result.
- Ask your lawyer about the most successful divorce cases he or she has handled. How many has he or she settled? Tried? Which does he or she prefer?
- If you don't like a lawyer, don't hire that lawyer; go find one you do like.

Prefiling Activities

- The most important part of the divorce is what happens before the papers are filed.

- You need a very good lawyer. Having hired one, you have to be honest with them and seek their advice.
- Seek advice about what's yours and what's not.
- Be prepared to lay out all the property you own, where it is, how much it is worth, and when it was acquired.
- In most states property acquired before marriage is separate property and does not have to be apportioned. In some states even though separate property is not apportioned between the spouses, it is considered in making the apportionment of other property.
- Do not attempt to hide assets.
- Do not sell your business to your brother for a dollar with the expectation of buying it back from him for 2 dollars after the divorce. Courts routinely unwind such transactions.
- Be meticulous and honest in your description of your assets and your spouse's assets.
- Get advice from your lawyer about what is rightfully yours and to what your spouse may have a rightful claim.
- Whatever amount your lawyer directs to be rightfully your property should be set aside.
- For example, if you have $2,000 in the savings account at the bank and the lawyer says you can have half of it, you should withdraw $1,000 and put it in a separate account.
- Remove your name and signature from the joint accounts. You do not want to be responsible if your spouse writes bad checks.
- Notify all your credit card companies that you want the account put in your name. If they will not do that, then close the account and open up different ones. You do not wish to be responsi-

ble if your soon-to-be-ex-spouse needs to buy new clothes or a sports car.

- Do not take everything, even if you are the breadwinner. If you take more than half, you look irresponsible to the court: What did you expect your spouse to do? Take half and the court knows you are a reasonable person.
- If possible, remove personal items, clothing, and other personal property from the residence (if you are moving out).
- If you are not moving out but your spouse is, then separate the property but do not damage it.

Protect Yourself
- Once the divorce is on file most states have a mechanism to protect the other spouse from threats of violence.
- If you are threatened, you must use these processes to protect yourself.
- Do not make threats against your spouse, and do not strike or hit your soon-to-be-ex. If you engage in violence, you could go to jail.
- If an action for an order of protection is filed against you, contest it. Even though you may ultimately have an order entered against you, you do not want the court to believe you are irresponsible.
- Keep in mind that in some states if there is an order of protection entered, you may have to hand over any firearms to law enforcement.
- Do not buy other firearms if you are a party to this kind of order.
- Violence is never an answer; it only makes the other questions more difficult to resolve.
- Taking action to set aside and safeguard property is important.

- If your spouse takes all the money in the joint checking and savings account, you might someday get it back.
- But you will not be able to hire a lawyer or pay your bills in the meantime.
- That's why prefiling activities are so very important.

Child Support Issues

- Child support is a fundamental right of every child.
- A child has a right to have the things he or she would have had but for the divorce.
- A child should not have to go without shoes, clothes, or food because one parent is trying to score points on the other.
- By the same token, the child is not entitled to a better lifestyle than he or she would have been entitled to.
- A good divorce lawyer can help you work out reasonable child support.
- Be prepared to pay a lot more child support than you believe you can afford if you indeed are going to pay child support.
- In most states the child support guidelines are published to make sure that the custodial parent gets the benefit of the doubt.
- Keep in mind that child support obligations in joint custody situations (where mom has the child Monday through Wednesday and dad has the child Thursday through Sunday) are often very minimal.

Maintenance

- Sometimes a non–wage-earning spouse may have no realistic way of making ends meet once a divorce is final. For example, he or she may have no marketable skills.

- In this situation the law sometimes provides for maintenance or what some courts call alimony.
- Alimony is usually limited and not given for life. Normally, someone gets alimony until he or she remarries, completes job training, or reaches a certain income threshold.
- If a spouse has a job or career and has the ability to make his or her own way in the world, then maintenance or alimony is rarely appropriate.

Modification
- It costs more to raise a teenager (who wants designer jeans) than it does to raise a child.
- When situations change, divorce decrees can often be modified.
- If $750 child support was fine in 1993 but is no longer meeting the needs of the child in 2007, then modification would be appropriate.
- Unless a divorce decree says it is not modifiable, it can be modified.
- Even a divorce decree that is not modifiable can be modified if the subject of the modification is child support.

Moving
- When a divorced parent must move to take a new job or go with a new spouse to a new location, it may drastically alter the relationship with the other spouse.
- Most states provide for a way to challenge any attempt by one spouse to take the children to a different state.

- Although sometimes these modifications are in everyone's best interest, the noncustodial spouse does have a right to be heard on the subject.

Enforcing Child Support

- It is unfortunate that some parents (both male and female) fail to live up to their child support obligations.
- The failure to live up to these obligations is sometimes based on the inability to pay.
- Often, the inability to pay excuse is just that, and courts do not give it much weight.
- If a spouse does not pay, every state has mechanisms to collect past due child support.
- In most cases, you don't need a lawyer to do this.
- You can use the state system to force the other party to pay back support.
- In some situations, federal tax returns can be intercepted.
- In other situations, you can get the district attorney in another state to file a motion to enforce the child support.
- The law that governs this is called the Uniform Reciprocal Enforcement of Support Act and has been enacted in most states.

Resources

- *Rebuilding: When Your Relationship Ends*, 3rd edition (Rebuilding Books; For Divorce and Beyond), by Bruce Fisher (Jan. 2005).
- *The Divorce Organizer and Planner,* by Brette McWhorter Sember (May 28, 2004).
- *Too Good to Leave, Too Bad to Stay: A Step-by-Step Guide to Help You Decide Whether to Stay*

In or Get Out of Your Relationship, by Mira Kirshenbaum (July 1, 1997).

- *The Complete Guide to Protecting Your Financial Security When Getting a Divorce*, by Alan Feigenbaum and Heather Linton (Mar. 19, 2004).
- Alliance for Non-Custodial Parents Rights (available online at http://www.ancpr.org/uifsa.html).
- Information on the Uniform Reciprocal Enforcement of Support Act, (available online at http://en.wikipedia.org/wiki/Uniform_Reciprocal_Enforcement_of_Support_Act).
- Divorce Source, a resource listing information for people considering divorce (available online at http://www.divorcesource.com).

Child Custody Law

Overview

Child custody is not a small thing. It is set aside here as a separate topic because it involves more issues than divorce. Child custody really asks this question: Between the mother and the father, who will do the best job of raising these children?

Sometimes it is not necessary to answer that question. If mom and dad both live and work in the same city, have extended family in the same location, and both have suitable homes for the children, then joint custody and joint physical custody may be the best approach for all parties.

Too often in divorce people act out of emotion and not intellect. In making a decision about whether to fight over custody, you have to ask the question, "What am I really fighting for?" If you are fighting because you wish to deprive your spouse of the children, you're fighting for the wrong reason. If you are fighting because you believe your spouse is not fit to be a parent, then, by all means, the fight is proper. But keep in mind that people often lie to themselves about this, and when they do, it costs them a lot of money.

Prevention

If I had a dollar for every person who called and asked for the name of the "meanest, nastiest, ugliest divorce attorney . . ." and then suggested that the sole quality necessary in their lawyer was a willingness to cause grief to the other side, I would be wealthy. Much of what goes on in custody cases is about evening scores and soothing bruised egos, and very little of it is about the welfare of the children.

The best prevention regarding custody is to be careful who you marry in the first place and to have zero tolerance for the kinds of behaviors that make people a bad parent. These include alcohol abuse, drug abuse, gambling, and other personality disorders. But sometimes love is blind and when the eyes open there are already children involved.

Documentation is the key in every child custody matter. To prevail in a child custody case, you must be able to show that the other party cannot meet his or her obligations as a parent, for example, drug abuse or gambling problems. Specific instances should be documented to prevail in a custody dispute.

Sometimes custody disputes break out between professionals. The attorney and the doctor who sue each other for custody have money to pour into the process but often lack the objectivity to realize that the process and the fight are themselves damaging to the children.

Whenever possible, joint custody is the best option.

Legal First Aid

The single most important thing you can do in getting custody is determine who the better parent is. Sometimes that means you have to document the things you do for your children. Other times it means you have to document what isn't done by the other party. But either way, it comes down to documentation.

Finding a Lawyer

- Talk to people who have recently been involved in custody maters.
- Talk frankly and up front about fees and retainers.
- A lawyer will usually want a retainer to cover costs for the first 6 months of the case. Some custody cases can be resolved quickly, but these are rare.

Custody Issues

- Most states have a mechanism for deciding custody issues at the outset of a case by placing the children with one spouse or the other.
- If custody of the children is an issue, then litigating this early and correctly is important. Have your lawyer get an early custody order that protects your rights.
- Only fight over custody if it matters.
- Custody fights are expensive, involve experts, and can easily reach the range of $50,000 where there are multiple allegations of wrongdoing.
- If joint custody is an option, it is almost always the absolute best option.
- In most cases that I have seen, people who fight over child custody are really doing no more than funding their lawyers' retirement accounts.
- Joint custody is the best solution for the children, and smart parents recognize that children should love both parents no matter where they live or whom they live with.
- For this reason, a fight over child custody is rarely if ever appropriate if joint custody can be awarded, except in those rare instances where there is child abuse.

- Unless you have photos, video, or good physical evidence of sexual abuse, do not make these claims in your divorce case.
- They are rarely more than a smokescreen for emotional blackmail.
- Courts see through this.
- More importantly, it becomes an expensive and arduous part of the divorce where no one wins but the child always loses.

Reasons for Custody

- Marital infidelity alone is not sufficient to deny custody to a mother or a father. Sometimes people fool around in their marriage; it doesn't make them bad parents.
- Drug abuse, alcohol abuse, and similar matters are grounds for seeking sole custody.
- Documentation is key.
- Keep in mind that some courts may allow a parent to get counseling.

Increased Burden for Men

- Although courts have made inroads in this area, men usually have a higher burden of proof in child custody cases than do women.
- This is because for many years the mother was the presumed custodian. Courts used to say there was a "tender years" presumption: during the "tender years" the child was thought to be better off with the mother. This is now no longer the law in most states, but the attitude still prevails in many courts.
- Therefore, men still have a much harder time getting sole custody of their children.
- To overcome this hurdle, you have to show, if you are challenging a mom, that she is not fit to care for the children.

- If there are DWI/DUI arrests, these play into the case.
- If there are witnesses who have seen the spouse drunk in front of the children, these play into the case.

Joint Custody

- Although men have a harder time getting sole custody, they often have a much easier time getting joint custody.
- This improves the amount of time the father gets with the child and, in some states, reduces the child support burden.
- Some states now presume that joint custody is proper and make any party wanting sole custody demonstrate why such an arrangement is better for the child.

Approach to Custody

- A good lawyer takes a measured approach to custody. Unless there is evidence of serious abuse or neglect, in most cases the lawyer will try to mediate custody and get a joint custody award.
- To truly fight about custody requires introducing evidence that is difficult to get legally. If you believe you have to follow your spouse to get the evidence, you should not do it. You should hire a professional investigator.
- You should only make a principled decision to fight for custody if the evidence is powerful and overwhelming. Otherwise, you take the chance on alienating the children of the marriage for a very long time.

What Judges Base Decisions On

- Today, it is the "best interest of the child" that controls how judges decide custody issues.

- This has been codified in the law of most states under § 402 of the Uniform Marriage and Divorce Act. That law provides as follows:

The court shall determine custody in accordance with the best interest of the child. The court shall consider all relevant factors including:

(1) The wishes of the child's parent or parents as to his custody;

(2) The wishes of the child as to his custodian;

(3) The interaction and interrelationship of the child with his parent or parents, his siblings, and any other person who may significantly affect the child's best interest;

(4) The child's adjustment to his home, school and community; and

(5) The mental and physical health of all individuals involved.

The court shall not consider conduct of a proposed custodian that does not affect his relationship to the child.

- In other words, what matters to a court doing its job properly is whether the decision it makes about custody ultimately benefits the child.

Interference With Custody and Visitation

- Sometimes when a court orders joint custody, it has to revisit the decision.
- When a parent precludes visitation by the other parent, it can be a change in circumstances that merits the court changing the custody arrangement.
- When a parent enters into a relationship that may be harmful to the child (for example, starts dating a person with a criminal record), it may affect the best interests of the child.
- When a parent who gets visitation routinely abuses it by keeping the children longer or by

not picking the child up at all, it too can create a serious change in circumstances mandating a change in custody.

Bottom Line

- Custody fights are always expensive, and unless there is a real risk of harm to the children, the children and the parties are almost always better off with joint custody arrangements.

Resources

- *Rebuilding: When Your Relationship Ends*, 3rd Edition (Rebuilding Books; For Divorce and Beyond), by Bruce Fisher (Jan. 2005).
- *The Divorce Organizer and Planner*, by Brette McWhorter Sember (May 28, 2004).
- *Too Good to Leave, Too Bad to Stay: A Step-by-Step Guide to Help You Decide Whether to Stay In or Get Out of Your Relationship*, by Mira Kirshenbaum (July 1, 1997).
- *The Complete Guide to Protecting Your Financial Security When Getting a Divorce*, by Alan Feigenbaum and Heather Linton (Mar. 19, 2004).
- Alliance for Non-Custodial Parents Rights (available online at http://www.ancpr.org/uifsa.html).
- Information on the Uniform Reciprocal Enforcement of Support Act (available online at http://en.wikipedia.org/wiki/Uniform_Reciprocal_Enforcement_of_Support_Act).
- Divorce Source, a resource listing information for people considering divorce (available online at http://www.divorcesource.com).

Conversion

■ Overview

Conversion is what happens when you take the use of a person's property from them. For example, a supervisor who takes away an employee's cellular phone because it rang during a meeting is, in effect, converting the phone from the employee's use to the supervisor's use. Conversion is a tort that permits a lawsuit when a person is deprived of the use of their property.

Similarly, if someone repossesses property (like a car or a house) and there is personal property inside, that property does not become the property of the repossessor or forecloser. Instead, it remains the property of the original owner (or possessor) of the vehicle. So although a repossessor has the right to seize a person's car if the bank so directs, the clothes and television set inside the car are still the property of the owner, not the bank.

Prevention

Conversion lawsuits arise when people mistakenly but under what lawyers call a "claim of right" take the use of property. For example, if a landlord drops by and finds a house he was renting vacant, except for a couch and sofa, he may believe the property has been abandoned. If he takes it and donates it to the Salvation Army, he may later find that he has "converted" the property and the tenant can sue for the value of the property.

Whenever you come into the possession of property that you do not know who the rightful owner is, most states have an "unclaimed property" statute that requires you to turn that property over to the state. You must follow this procedure to legally claim an interest in that property later or to be free of someone's conversion claim.

Legal First Aid

- If you find property, turn it in.
- If someone abandons property on your land, you should follow the unclaimed property statute.
- In some jurisdictions you must run a newspaper advertisement to notify the owner of the property, even if you don't know who it is.
- If property has a title (e.g., car, boat, trailer), there may be specific statutes that permit you to sell the property (or salvage the property), but you must comply with the state's rules. If you fail to, you could be sued.
- If someone takes your property unlawfully, first make a demand to have the property returned.
- If someone refuses your demand, you have the right to file a "replevin" lawsuit to get the property back.

Resources

- Unclaimed Property Page (available online at http://www.kantrowitz.com/kantrowitz/uncl-prop.html).

Landlord–Tenant

▇ Overview

At some point in most people's lives they are forced to rent property. Renters become subject to the conditions imposed by the landlord, and a subset of law called Landlord–Tenant Law governs the relationship between these parties.

In many cases landlords and tenants get along fine. They rarely if ever have issues as long as the rent is paid and the house or apartment remains in good working order. When they do not, issues arise between the parties. This section deals with problems of renters and problems of landlords in separate sections.

Prevention

Few people bother to keep a copy of the lease they sign when they rent an apartment or house, yet it often is the most important document they have. This is because so frequently the lease controls what rights they have and what remedies they can use.

For the landlord, a well-worded lease with proper language and protections limits the risks of renting property to a tenant. To a tenant, a good lease provides information about what's expected of them and what the landlord will take care of.

Sometimes a lease is badly written, containing provisions that are clearly unlawful. Other times the leases are written in such a way that the landlord gives up valuable rights.

Whether you are a landlord or a tenant, the lease is the most important document you have and governs your relationship. You should make an extra effort to ensure that it is a good document.

Legal First Aid

For Renters on Renting

- Talk to other tenants. Make sure they are happy. If they are not, rent somewhere else.
- Check out the security situation. Is the property secure? Are there secure locks on the doors? Is hallway lighting adequate and access to hallways controlled?
- Check out the local sex offender list on the Internet. Are any child predators or sexual criminals living in the vicinity?
- Get references. You can be sure the landlord is checking you out. Check him or her out, too.
- Go to the courthouse and see if anyone has sued this landlord or company. If so, contact them and find out what the problems were.
- If you are given a lease, take it to a lawyer if you don't understand everything it says.
- Make sure that all utilities are apportioned by meter. Never agree to split one type of metered utility (like gas or electric) with another tenant or to pay a fixed sum for this to the landlord.
- The lease governs the relationship between you and the landlord; you want to make sure that it protects you from any failures by the landlord.
- Beware of arbitration clauses. If a lease provides that the landlord can sue you but that you

have to arbitrate any claims against the landlord, you don't want to live there.
- Keep a copy of your lease in a safe place.
- Make sure the landlord has insurance. Buy a
  renter's insurance policy of your own. This is
  very important if you want to protect your stuff
  from being stolen.

For Renters With Problems

- If you have problems with your landlord, talk to
  him or her first.
- If the landlord does not repair problems in your
  home, send him or her written notice that you
  intend to make the repairs and deduct the
  charges from the rent. Give the landlord a date
  and you are certain to get the problem fixed.
  Send the letter by certified mail, and keep a
  copy of the receipt.
- If the landlord fails to make the repairs, you
  can also threaten to breach the lease if the les-
  sor does not keep the property maintained.
  Rather than doing repairs, you can simply
  move if you want to in that situation.
- Take photos of all problems.
- Make and keep a record of any conversations
  you have with the landlord about any problems.
- Records and photos are what are necessary if the
  landlord sues you later for breaching the lease.
- Usually, a landlord will make repairs if you
  simply let him or her know of the problems.
- If the landlord does not make repairs, you have
  what is called a "breach of the warranty of hab-
  itability" if the unrepaired problem (e.g., lack of
  heat) makes it hard for you to remain there.
- If a landlord insists on dropping by and inspect-
  ing your property without notice and at odd

times, you should check your lease. Most leases require that the landlord give notice. If the landlord does not give notice, he or she is breaching the "covenant of quiet enjoyment" that comes with your property.

- It is rarely worthwhile to stay in a property where you have to make repairs and deduct them from the rent. You should simply breach the lease and move in most cases.
- If you do breach the lease, make sure there are multiple witnesses to the problems with the leased premises in the event the case needs to be heard in court.

For Landlords on Renting

- Check out the tenant.
- Run a full credit check.
- If you do not have a credit check capability, at least check your local court records.
- If possible, run a criminal background check on your tenants.
- Check the sex offender registry. The lovely 30-year-old woman may very well be a sex offender.
- Insist on deposits in cash or certified checks and give receipts.
- Take checks for rent only, and if you've received a bad check from a tenant, require future payments by money order or certified funds.
- A tenant may issue a bad check and move in, and then the landlord either has to forego getting the deposit or evict the tenant, which costs him or her even more money.
- Do not ever let a renter have possession on the basis of a personal or business check unless you have personally cleared the check through the bank.

- Once a tenant is in a property, it is very hard to remove them.

General Landlord Issues

- Property must be kept in a safe condition.
- Lighting must be proper for the common areas and deter criminal activity.
- Warnings should be posted in all public areas.
- Make sure you have adequate insurance to cover the property and your risk.
- Make sure your insurance covers negligent acts by employees.
- Property in a high-crime area should be sold. You do not wish to become an insurer of your property's safety.
- Door locks must be secure and must safeguard the tenant's premises.
- Keys (particularly master keys) should be secured and their use limited to bonded employees.
- Never hire a maintenance person or other employee without a criminal background check. Always adhere to immigration law and the rules regarding hiring citizens or aliens.
- Assume that where there is smoke, there is fire. If tenants complain about the manager being abusive, you should probably make changes in your staff.

For Landlords With Problems

- When a tenant becomes a problem, the first step is to ask him or her to leave.
- Do not let a tenant get more than 2 weeks late with rent before taking action.
- A tenant who fails to pay rent on time should never have his or her lease renewed.
- A tenant may not always leave when his or her lease is up. It is always wise to send formal

notices of eviction to tenants whose lease is expiring and will not be renewed.

- Never store property for a tenant in some other part of your facility unless you are willing to insure it.

Resources

- *Renters Resource, Landlord–Tenant Problems: Self-Help Guide*, by Patricia Williams (July 30, 1999).
- *What Every Landlord Needs to Know: Time and Money-Saving Solutions to Your Most Annoying Problems*, by Richard H. Jorgensen (Aug. 1, 2004).
- *The Good, the Bad, and Evictions: A Layman's Guide to Residential Landlord and Tenant Problems*, by J. G. Hardy (1998).
- *Landlord and Tenant Practice: The Problem Tenant*, by Kenneth A. Krems (2000).
- *Every Tenant's Legal Guide*, by Janet Portman and Marcia Stewart (Apr. 30, 2007).

Consumer Fraud

Overview

Consumer fraud produces billions in profits every year for shady operators and costs citizens millions in every state in the union. Although everyone is familiar with the "free travel" and "free vacation" scams run by telemarketers out of boiler rooms in Florida and elsewhere, lots of consumer fraud happens every day of the year in broad daylight, out in the open.

Consumer fraud is the use of artifice, deception, trickery, deceit, or the omission of key facts to sell a product. In the 1950s, magazines and newspapers like *Grit* and the *National Enquirer* had hundreds of classified advertisements that offered work-from-home or other schemes guaranteed to make money for the bored and lonely reader. One scam in particular offered to sell a "copper engraving" of Abraham Lincoln, the "Great Emancipator" for $19.95. When people sent in their money they would often receive their copper engraving by return mail, in an envelope. The envelope would contain one U.S. penny.

With the Internet and e-Bay it is now even easier to separate the gullible from their money. Anyone who does business on the Internet knows that the chance of your identity being stolen rises every time you do business with a merchant and provide credit card information.

Consumer fraud involves credit card companies charging more interest than permitted by law; it involves insurance companies collecting premiums or premium increases unlawfully. The list of companies from Apple to Wachovia who have been sued in class action consumer fraud litigation is long and extensive.

Prevention

The best way to prevent becoming a victim of consumer fraud, and this is not rocket science, is to realize that everything that sounds too good to be true probably is. A 5-day vacation for four people for $375 sounds too good to be true. By the time you pay the booking fees and the insurance and the other 14 charges the company adds on, your $375 vacation has cost you $1,500. If you deal with local, reputable merchants that you've dealt with previously or whom others have recommended, you are rarely going to get burned.

The key to avoiding consumer fraud is to know the company you're dealing with, read the material carefully, and ask questions if anything sounds too good to be true. Deal with people you know, as mentioned earlier. When you have to deal with an agency or entity that you've not previously dealt with, get references and learn all you can about the organization before calling them. Don't be afraid to ask questions. Never buy anything until you are convinced that you're dealing with an honest company.

Legal First Aid

- If you've had the wool pulled over your eyes, do the following:

- Send a letter, by fax if possible, to the company. Explain the problem and demand a refund. Give the company a deadline in which to respond. If they fail to do so, you take the next step.
- Contact the consumer fraud division of the Attorney General's office in your state and file a formal complaint.

- In some cases, you may want to also file a complaint with the Federal Trade Commission.
- If neither the Attorney General nor the Federal Trade Commission can assist you with getting your money back, contact a lawyer.
- If the amount of money is small (less than $3,000 in most states), you can sue the company in small claims court.
- All you have to show is that the company used a deceptive advertisement or communication to take your money and gave you less than you bargained for (or charged you more than you promised to pay).
- You may have been ripped off without even knowing it. Many times class action lawsuits are filed on your behalf and you do not receive notice of these actions. There are services where you can check to see if a company you routinely do business with has been sued (visit http://www.classactionworld.com).

Resources

- *The Art of the Steal: How to Protect Yourself and Your Business from Fraud, America's #1 Crime*, by Frank W. Abagnale (Jan. 29, 2002).
- *Under Investigation: The Inside Story of the Florida Attorney General's Investigation of Wilhelmina Scouting Network, the Largest Model*

and Talent Scam in America, by Les Henderson (Sep. 12, 2006).

- *Gotcha Capitalism: How Hidden Fees Rip You Off Every Day—and What You Can Do About It*, by Bob Sullivan (Jan. 18, 2008).
- Listing of consumer-based class action lawsuits (available online at http://www.classaction world.com).

Domestic Violence

Overview

Domestic violence and emotional abuse are control behaviors. In other words, the threats of violence, the use of violence, or the use of emotionally charged words are used by one person in a relationship to control the other person. Although it is often thought of in terms of male violence directed against females in a marital relationship, the truth is that it crosses lines of gender, race, education, and ethnicity. It is every person's right to be free from violence or threats of violence.

Domestic violence can be criminal. Whether violence is physical or verbal and whether the violence is witnessed or leaves evidence of contact often determines whether police or other agencies are willing to get involved. Although emotional, psychological, and financial abuse are not usually criminal behaviors, they often lead to criminal violence. Domestic violence is a plague.

Whereas anyone can be a victim, in most cases the weakest parties in a relationship are the most common ones. Women and children are more commonly abused by bigger and stronger males, although many times women give as good as they get in a domestic relationships. Police officers are trained not to assume that domestic violence starts with the man.

Like most forms of violence, domestic violence often arises out of substance abuse, particularly alcohol abuse. Alcohol is more often than not a precipitating factor in family violence and may be at the root of the relationship problems.

Sometimes spouses seeking a tactical advantage in divorce litigation make false allegations of domestic violence. This is covered in "Assertions of Domestic Violence That Are Untrue," found later in this chapter.

Prevention

The best way to prevent domestic violence is to be watchful and careful in developing relationships in the first place. Individuals who hit, or who threaten to hit, are often suffering from behaviors learned as children. Parents who hit them got what they wanted, and now they know if they inflict violence on others, most of the time they get what they want. The key to understanding domestic violence is that it is about control. And sadly, most abusers are clueless about why they do what they do. In most cases abusers simply say that this is the way they were brought up. Because violence is a learned behavior, individuals who display that behavior are people to be avoided in forming relationships.

If you find yourself in a domestic relationship and you have a partner who is violent, seek counseling. Often, if you and your partner can get help, you can break the cycle of violence. But if a partner will not seek help or will not accept help, then you have to act to protect yourself, and that means leaving the relationship.

Legal First Aid

Domestic Violence Against You

- You have options. This is not the 1950s. Even if your spouse controls the money and the car keys, you can find help in your community to break free from the cycle of violence.
- Your personal safety, and that of any children, is the predominant concern in any domestic violence situation.
  - Children are often silent victims.
  - They not only suffer abuse themselves, they see the abuse inflicted on one of the spouses and internalize that abuse themselves.
  - Even if you don't act to protect yourself, you must act to protect your children.
- If you have a partner who is violent, you need to get out of the relationship if they are unwilling to change.
- Never accept an abuser's promise not to abuse; they don't mean to break it, but they will.
- Unless and until an abuser gets help, do not go back into the relationship.
- Most abusers don't like the idea of you asserting control over your own life and often act out more violently when you announce plans to leave. For this reason, never announce the plans, just leave.
- Because abusers are master manipulators, they may try everything in the world, including pleading, to get you to change your mind. Do not do it.
- Most states have methods to obtain a personal order of protection that requires the abuser to avoid contact with you. Insist on getting such an order from the local court.

- In most states you do not need a lawyer.
- In most states there is not a filing fee.
- You have to tell the judge why you are afraid of the other party.
- There is a hearing on the order in 10 days where the other side can contest the issuance of the order.
- If the order is violated, prosecute.
- Abusers rely on your willingness to be controlled, and your desire not to cause trouble, and may try to convince you not to prosecute violations or to drop such an order.
- Under no circumstances should you do so.
- If your partner has firearms or weaponry, always get an order of protection. Domestic issues make people do crazy things.

Assertions of Domestic Violence That Are Untrue

- If you are accused of domestic violence, it is imperative that you retain an attorney and fight the allegations.
- Allegations of domestic violence, if believed by a court, can affect your ability to retain your own possessions, can affect the property settlement, and may impact your rights as a custodial or noncustodial parent.
- An allegation of abuse is not proof of abuse. Retain an attorney who has handled a prior case where there were false allegations.
- It may be necessary to involve neighbors, friends, and coworkers to establish that there was no abuse. You should get witnesses who can tell the court the following:
  - They never found you to be abusive.
  - You have never hit your partner in their presence.

- Coworkers should testify that the spouse has not come to work with bruises or injuries.
- Because allegations of abuse have an effect on the community, your efforts are aimed at protecting your reputation.
- Some professionals, like law enforcement agents and police officers, who are required to carry weapons on duty, may be forced to defend these accusations to retain their positions as police officers.
- Health care workers convicted of domestic violence (or who have orders of protection entered against them) may be disqualified from working with elderly patients in some states.
- If a false allegation has been leveled against a clinician, it is vital to defend against that and to employ an attorney with experience in defending these allegations.

Resources

- Online resource for domestic violence (available online at www.domesticviolence.org).
- *Why Does He Do That?: Inside the Minds of Angry and Controlling Men*, by Lundy Bancroft (Sop. 2, 2003).
- *Surviving Domestic Violence: Voices of Women Who Broke Free*, by Elaine Weiss (Feb. 2004).
- *Healing the Trauma of Domestic Violence: A Workbook for Women* (New Harbinger Self-Help Workbook), by Edward S. Kubany, Mari A. McCaig, and Janet R. Laconsay (Aug. 2004).
- *Handbook of Domestic Violence Intervention Strategies: Policies, Programs, and Legal Remedies*, by Albert R. Roberts and Marjory D. Fields (Mar. 28, 2002).

Negligence-Based Torts

▪ Overview

In 2006 there were more than 38,000 fatal vehicle accidents, and, according to the Fatality Analysis Reporting System, that number has stayed about the same since 1994. In addition to automobile accidents, almost every kind of passenger vehicle carries with it the possibility of an injury. Although not all injuries are the responsibility of someone else, many are, and the tort law system exists to place the burden of paying for negligence on the people who have the greatest incentive to be careful, which are the people operating their vehicles in an unsafe manner.

In addition to vehicular accidents, people walk onto land occupied by others and suffer accidents because of dangerous conditions. For example, a sidewalk may be cracked, leading to a fall and a broken hip. A supermarket floor may be wet and slippery, leading to the same result. A neighbor's dog might bite. A well dug years earlier and not carefully covered may result in a drowning. All these situations are cases where the injured party or their family may recover.

Prevention

The first step in protecting yourself and your assets from liability is to obtain good insurance for anything you drive or operate, including tractors, lawnmowers, and golf carts. In addition, even if you rent, you should have some form of liability insurance for your personal property that carries with it protection against things that may not be easily foreseen. For example, a dog who has never bitten a soul may well attack a small child for reasons clear only to the dog. When something like that happens, if you do not have liability insurance, you could subject yourself to liability that might force you into bankruptcy.

Insurance does more than provide you with a fund to pay damages. It provides you with an attorney loyal only to you who defends you against these actions. By the same token, you should never ride in a car that is not insured. You should never deal with a business that is uninsured. You should never operate a business without insurance.

Legal First Aid

You Are Injured by Negligence in an Auto Accident

- Do not make any statements at the scene.
- Seek medical aid if necessary. Every motor vehicle accident involving damage to a vehicle, no matter how slight, should cause everyone in the vehicle to be checked out by an emergency room physician or their family doctor.
- Often, signs of injury are not immediately apparent, particularly when the injury is to soft tissue, like the musculature of the back or neck.
- Do not give a statement to any adjuster (yours or anyone else's) until you have talked to an attorney.
- Do not give any statements to police officers or adjusters at the hospital. Tell them you must wait to talk to them until you are well enough

to give a statement. If you are sick enough to be in the hospital, you are too sick to talk to investigators.

- Go to your regular doctor. Do not ask an attorney for a recommendation on a physician. This makes it look like you're trying to game the system.
- If you are seriously injured, your family should contact an attorney immediately.
- An investigation of the accident or injury focusing on what was at the scene and the conditions at the date and time of the accident is the most important part of any tort case.
- As soon as you are in a condition to do it, write down everything that happened on a piece of paper and label it "Notes Prepared for My Attorney" (see Appendix 1).
- Contact an attorney who handles accident and injury cases for plaintiffs.
- Do not talk with anyone about your case other than your attorney.
- Do get the names of witnesses who may have seen what happened.
- Do get a copy of the report of the accident filed by any police agency.
- Keep the vehicle, even if totaled in the accident, until it can be determined if there is a claim against the automaker.

Other Negligence

- Make a complete record of what happened.
- Take photographs of the property if property was involved.
- If you cannot get photographs of the property without going back onto the land where the accident occurred, wait for your attorney to get the photographs.

- Make a drawing of what the scene looked like, if possible, and diagram everything.
- Make a list of witnesses.
- Get copies of all ambulance reports and any medical records regarding treatment you received.
- If a 911 call was involved, notify the police agency promptly to get a copy because these are often lost after 48 to 72 hours.

Someone Is Hurt on Your Property

- Obtain medical aid first by calling 911 and then provide first aid until paramedics or other medical staff arrive.
- If you were not involved in the injury (i.e., you did nothing that caused the incident), give investigating officers a statement of what you saw and when you saw it.
- Make a record of what happened.
- Take photographs of the accident scene immediately after investigators leave.
- Contact your insurance agent and report the incident to him or her.

Someone Claims You Are/Were Negligent

- Do not give any adjuster or investigator a statement until you have contacted an attorney.
- Contact your insurance company for instructions.
- Your attorney will usually not let you speak to adjusters or others.
- As soon as possible, write down everything that happened on a piece of paper and label it "Notes Prepared for My Attorney" (see Appendix 1).
- Review your notes and make sure they are as complete as they can be.
- Once finished, put them away and do not edit them further.

- Do not talk to friends or acquaintances about what happened.
- Do not "tell your story" to other people. The more times other people hear it, the more errors there will be in what they remember about what you said.
- Do not try to be your own lawyer. Hire a good attorney and trust him or her to represent you. Sometimes people get the idea that paying an attorney just means less money for them. Sixty-five percent of a $100,000 settlement is more money than 100% of a $30,000 settlement.
- Do make a list of witnesses.
- Get a copy of any 911 tape if possible.
- Get the names of all people who responded to the accident.

Resources

- Nolo Press Traffic Accident FAQ (available online at http://www.nolo.com/article.cfm/object Id/6B2EE6CB-05E3-4F51-A5CC59140D47D021 /catID/CF015A63-6B69-4EED-A34B6F40 35C8BE0E/104/263/FAQ).
- What To Do After an Accident, California State Bar (available online at http://www.calbar.ca .gov/state/calbar/calbar_extend.jsp?cid=10581 &id=2174).

Strict Liability-Based Torts

▪ Overview

There are some things that no matter what happens, they cannot be made safe. For this reason the law places a duty of strict liability on the person who engages in the activity to provide for the safety of others. Electrical power lines are one area where the law imposes strict liability on the utility if anyone is injured as a result of the overhead lines falling.

Strict liability also includes liability for failure to warn of a device's dangerous propensities. For example, if a lawnmower might cause hearing damage because of the loud motor, the maker needs to warn of it. If someone uses a product without being warned of the dangers and suffers an adverse result, then the product manufacturer is liable.

Similarly, if you keep a non-native or wild and dangerous animal, you are responsible if it gets out and injures someone. Certain animals, like pit bull terriers, are considered so dangerous that the law imposes strict liability on anyone keeping such an animal. The same would be true for the pet cobra or pet rattlesnake.

Strict liability means that the person with the dangerous product, device, or animal is charged with preventing, as much as possible, any harm that might arise out of the activity in which they engage.

Prevention

It is beyond the scope of this pocket book to advise manufacturers on this line of liability. As a consumer you should always exercise care around utilities and in the conduct of your daily activities. If you are injured as a result of a dangerous condition on property or because of a defective product, you should follow the steps below and see an attorney as quickly as possible.

Legal First Aid

Injuries to Self or Family

- Do not make any statements at the scene where you or a loved one is injured.
- Keep all evidence relating to any product. Do not discard the defective product.
- Do not give a statement to any adjuster (yours or anyone else's) until you have talked to an attorney.
- Seek medical aid when necessary.
- If you are seriously injured, your family should contact an attorney immediately to begin an investigation.
- An investigation of the accident or injury focusing on what was at the scene and the conditions at the time of the incident causing the injuries.
- A complete record of what happened should be made on a piece of paper and labeled "Notes Prepared for My Attorney" (see Appendix 1).
- Do not talk with anyone about your case other than your attorney.
- Do get the names of witnesses who may have seen what happened.

- Take photographs of the property if property was involved.
- If you cannot get photographs of the property without going back onto the land where the incident occurred, wait for your attorney to get the photographs.
- Make a drawing of what the scene looked like, if possible, and diagram everything.
- Make a list of witnesses and diagram where they were standing.
- Get copies of all ambulance reports and any medical records regarding treatment you received.
- If a 911 call was involved, notify the police agency promptly to get a copy because these are often lost after 48 to 72 hours.

Your Animal or a Product You Sold Causes Injury
- Contact your insurer immediately.
- Do not speak to anyone until you talk to an attorney.
- Do not make a written statement.
- Do not talk to the other party's adjuster or insurance company.
- Do not talk to the other party's lawyer.
- Take photographs if possible and practical.
- Trust your attorney to handle the matter.

Resources
- Defective and Dangerous Products at FindLaw (available online at http://injury.findlaw.com/defective-dangerous-products/defectivedang erous-products-faq).

Property Damage Claims

▇ Overview

When we buy property, we often buy it with the idea that we'll reside on it for the rest of our lives in peace and in harmony with our neighbors. But sometimes neighbors buy property with different ideas. They want to put up a go-cart track. They want to start a hog-farming operation. They want to smelt lead. When property is destroyed or rendered less valuable by the actions of others, nuisance and trespass law are often the area where lawyers provide assistance.

Prevention

Usually, the best guarantee against someone damaging your use of property or interfering with your business use of property is to have the property properly zoned at the outset. When you do this, you ensure that the use of the property will fit in with the local area, and you have government approval for what you are doing. However, even that is no guarantee that your property use will not affect someone else. If you make changes to your property that affect the way the property drains rainwater, for example, and flood out a neighbor in the process, you might be liable for the result.

For this reason any change in property use needs to be measured against the needs of your neighbors, and good communication at the front end often means no problems on the back end. However, not all people are reasonable in the use of their land or in your use of your land, and you may need to hire a lawyer if someone trespasses on your land or if you inadvertently create a nuisance on someone else's.

Legal First Aid

Trespass

- Trespass is unauthorized entry onto land.
- It can be caused by walking or driving across someone's land or by putting something on someone's land.
- A business may trespass on a neighbor's property, for example, by allowing its waste products to be blown (or run off during rains) onto the property.
- Trespass can be compensated by damages or stopped by an injunction.
- An injunction is a court order to stop the trespass that carries with it specific penalties if violated.

Nuisance

- When someone uses his or her property in a way that causes damages to others, he or she is creating a nuisance.
- For example, a property owner in a residential neighborhood who opens an outdoor shooting range might well create a nuisance.
- A property owner who allowed his or her property to be used by criminals (for the manufac-

ture of drugs, as one example) might be creating a nuisance.

- Under nuisance laws the court can order damages to remedy the harm done to the plaintiff (usually the diminishment of property values), or it can order an injunction.
- An injunction is a court order to stop the activities creating a nuisance. It carries with it specific penalties if violated.

Resources

- Trespass Law (available online at http://en .wikipedia.org/wiki/Trespass_to_land).

Legal First Aid for a Criminal Law Problem

Introduction to Legal First Aid for a Criminal Law Problem

8

In the pages that follow the most common criminal matters arising in health care are discussed and specific advice about specific criminal charges are offered. However, some general advice applies to all criminal matters. These are the things you absolutely must know when dealing with any kind of investigator whether from the city, county, state, or federal government.

At the outset, this book presumes that a person reading it is not guilty of a crime, just the way the Constitution presumes that you are innocent until proved guilty. What follows is not a treatise for the guilty individual to follow to avoid sanction. That is not its purpose. Its purpose is to help the person who is in the wrong place at the wrong time. The person who did not do anything wrong but who circumstances suggest might be guilty of doing something wrong. I have no intent to obstruct a legitimate investigation into wrongdoing. A lawyer's job is to presume his or her client is not guilty and make the state or federal government prove its case.

In the pages that follow we look first at the criminal acts for which federal and state authorities can prosecute. After explaining the crimes we focus on how to avoid such situations and how to prevent getting caught up in the investigative process.

In dealing with criminal matters, the legal first aid is all the same. It is captured in the section immediately following this one. If there is a criminal law problem and you need immediate first aid for that problem, read that material first.

■ The Right to Remain Silent

The right to not answer questions posed by investigators is enshrined in the Constitution. With the exception of "enemy combatants," everyone has the right to refuse to be questioned, and the right is actually more fundamental than that. Once you tell the police or investigative officers that you do not wish to be questioned, they cannot question you.

The fact is that most innocent people want to talk to the police. They view their role as being there to help the police catch the "bad guy." As high-profile cases like the JonBenet Ramsey case made clear, sometimes that desire to help the police solve a crime tends to make them look guilty in the absence of specific facts establishing their guilt. So, although it might seem counterintuitive for an individual who has done nothing wrong to refuse to speak to the police or federal investigators, often that is the best thing they can do.

Sometimes a law enforcement person may legitimately seek witness statements from people who saw what happened. But sometimes they use this as a ploy to get information out of someone they suspect of doing something bad. A person not schooled in interrogation might never understand the difference until they have said things that made them look guilty. In a recent case I had an individual who was asked how many text messages he sent to a person. He considered "conversations" and not individual text message units and vastly underestimated the number he had sent. The police charged him with statutory rape because he did not give them an accurate number.

Often investigators use one of two ploys to get people to talk after they have invoked their right to remain silent. The first is what I call the "innocent person" strategy. The police suggest that if you are innocent you should have nothing to hide and that only a guilty person would invoke their right to remain silent. Police are trained to believe this. They are also trained to manipulate people. Their job is to get a conviction. And, unfortunately, as recent cases demonstrate, sometimes police officers follow the wrong leads and the wrong suspects while the guilty go free. As a result, sometimes innocent people who had "nothing to hide" find out that talking to the investigators is never in their best interest. Sadly, they discover this too late. If an investigator attempts to browbeat you into holding a conversation, tell him or her that you will not say anything more.

The second strategy interrogators use is to say "fine, you don't have to talk, but you have to listen to me." Technically, this is not true. Once you tell them you do not want to be questioned, they have to leave you alone. They cannot interrogate you under the guise of "informing you." The investigators intentionally say things that are not true either to get a rise out of you or to get information from you. For example, they might say, "your coworkers saw you take Diprivan from the Pyxis system." The purpose of this is to get you to say "I never took anything out of the Pxyis system." Once they engage you and you start responding to them, they can and often will attempt to confuse and mislead you. For example, they might say, "Oh really, then why do you have a Pyxis ID in the system? Are you saying you never used this equipment?" Of course, now you feel compelled to clarify your earlier answer. "When I said never, I meant I never did what you said I did." Frequently, two investigators will team up, playing good cop and bad cop and before long your right to remain silent has been violated without you even knowing it.

Once you invoke your right to remain silent, do not rise to any bait or any suggestions by investigators. Do not speak, and do not listen to investigators after that point.

■ The Right to Counsel

Also enshrined in the Constitution is the right to counsel. Even if you cannot afford a lawyer, you can have one appointed. Always, and under every circumstance, demand a lawyer if you are questioned or if an investigator asks to "interview" you.

The lawyer's job is to keep things fair. His or her job is to make certain that you do not answer questions like "when did you stop beating your wife?" The lawyer's job is to protect you from investigators who might want you to say things you shouldn't say.

Usually, it is in the client's best interest to give no interviews. Sometimes, however, situations present where if the client does not agree to an interview, bad things happen. Recently, I represented a teacher accused of a sex crime. The teacher was not guilty of anything other than sending text messages to the student. But the student had made a false accusation of sexual conduct, and even though the accusation had not been reported at the time and was only reported 18 months later, the police still investigated. The following is from the transcript of the interview:

Investigator: So why would this girl say these things about you?

Client: I don't know.

Investigator: You taught her, you must know how she thinks. I mean, you taught her how to think didn't you. About some things?

Client: I taught her math. I helped her with her homework.

Investigator: Homework assigned by other teachers, not by you?

Client: She wasn't in my class, but she seemed to understand things better with me than some of the other teachers. She and I communicated very well.

Investigator: So if anyone would know why she would make these charges, it ought to be you. You two communicated so well and all.

Lawyer: Stop right there. I am not going to let you ask my client to speculate on what this girl's state of mind is. He told you he didn't know what her state of mind was or why she would do this. Let it go.

Investigator: So you tell me, why would she say this if it wasn't true? I'm thinking it is true, and that's why you don't want to answer my question.

Lawyer: OK, that's strike two. That's the same question. The next question on this topic will be your last. If you have other relevant questions, ask them, otherwise we're done here.

Attorneys who are good at what they do keep clients from saying things or being dragged into conversations they do not want to have. In the example above, the police officer is trying to get the client to say the victim is lying. On the stand, in the court, the police officer can later say that the client called the purported victim a liar. Without an attorney to keep the questions honest, the investigator's notes will reflect a completely different spin on the conversations. For that reason, never consent to an interview without counsel.

▌ The Right to Choose Time and Place

Police officers often show up unannounced at the door on a Friday night with a badge and a gun and want to talk to you right then. They may want you to "take a ride downtown" so they can conduct the interview in a location where they control when and where you can go and what you can do. Unless you are under arrest, you have the right to say no, and you should. First, it is almost never a good idea to talk to police. But, if you and your attorney decide to speak to them, do it on your terms. The best time to talk about something is after you have reviewed the matter, contacted counsel, found out what is at issue, and have had time to reflect on and recollect the events at issue.

You can schedule a time and place for the interview. I recommend having the investigators come to the lawyer's office, where they are out of their element and where if they do not behave themselves they can be asked to leave. An interview at a police station, where clients often do not feel free to leave, is much more emotionally exhausting than the same interview at a lawyer's office.

▌ If You Are Arrested

If police or federal agents place you under arrest, they believe they have sufficient evidence to hold you for a crime. In that situation there is only one right response. First, call an attorney and do not do or say anything to anyone until he or she tells you that you can. Second, do not consent to an interview. Invoke your right to counsel and invoke your right to remain silent.

▌ Conclusion

If you take nothing else away from this book, make sure you understand this: When police are talking to you, they are not your friend. They cannot ever make things better for you; they can only make them worse. Cooperation may have its time and place, if indeed you did something wrong. But that is a decision for a lawyer to make, based on the evidence and after reflection. It is not something that you should do in the heat of the moment.

▌ Legal First Aid: Read This First

- You have the right to remain silent.
- You have the right to speak with an attorney.
- Anything you say to investigators or anyone else may be used against you.
- You have a right not to be questioned.
- No jury may be told that you exercised your right to remain silent.

These are important rights guaranteed by the U.S. Constitution. They are not designed to protect guilty people. They are designed to protect innocent people. When you exercise your rights under the Constitution, you are exercising rights that the founding fathers thought were important enough to die for. If you ignore these rights, you do so at your peril.

There are only two absolutes any time a criminal inquiry starts. The first absolute is that you remain silent until you have spoken to an attorney. The second is that you absolutely need an attorney. The police have an attorney (the district attorney). The FBI has an attorney (the U.S. Attorney). There is nothing wrong with you having an attorney. Asking for an attorney does not make you look guilty. It makes you look like a smart person. Do not under any circumstances fall for the lie that if you are innocent you do not need a lawyer. If you are innocent, you definitely need a lawyer.

Under our system of justice you do not have to admit guilt. The state has to prove guilt beyond a reasonable doubt and without any of your words being used against you. If you are innocent the last thing you want to do is give the authorities an excuse to prosecute you because you said something stupid. That's why the two "absolutes" of silence and counsel go hand in hand.

With these rights and observations in mind, whenever there is a criminal inquiry, these points should guide you:

- Politely inform any investigator who approaches you to ask questions that you will not speak with them until your attorney is present.
  - When you ask to contact an attorney you are likely to hear the following responses from investigators:
    - We are not interested in you.
      - I understand, but because you have attorneys that advise you, I want an attorney to advise me.
    - This doesn't concern your conduct.
      - I understand, but I want an attorney's advice on what questions to answer and what questions not to answer.
    - If you're innocent, you don't need an attorney.
      - I am innocent, and that's exactly why I need an attorney.
    - We are interested in what you know and what you told your employer, not in anything you did or didn't do.
      - Because this involves my employer, I want my employer's general counsel involved in the interview. I don't

> want you getting me in trouble
> with the boss.

- You do not owe an investigator any response,
  however. You do not have to debate whether
  you need an attorney and you do not have to
  prove you need one. You just have to tell them
  you will not be talked to without one.
- Do this even if you are not the target of the investigation.
  - You could easily open your mouth and
    make yourself a target of the investigation.
- Without an attorney to help you marshal the
  facts and keep you answering only appropriate
  questions, you might be tricked into saying
  something that incriminates you.
- It bears repeating: *Contact an attorney imme-
  diately.*
  - Do not engage in conversation with the in-
    vestigator until an attorney is present.
  - Again, you do not need to provide an expla-
    nation for why you need an attorney.
  - If you must provide this explanation, tell
    the investigator to read the Sixth Amend-
    ment to the U.S. Constitution and the
    Supreme Court decision in *Miranda v. Ari-
    zona.*
- Once an attorney is present, meet privately
  with him or her.
- Make sure the attorney has all the information
  about the situation the investigator is inter-
  ested in.
- *Do not consent to anything.* Among the things
  the authorities may ask your consent to are the
  following:
  - *Do not consent to* a search of any of your
    personal property including your:

- Home
- Locker
- Car
- Boat
- Personal effects
- Blood work
- DNA samples
- Hair samples
  - *Do not consent to* appearing in a "lineup."
  - *Do not consent to* the use of your photograph in a photo lineup.
  - *Do not consent to* access to your bank accounts or bank statements.
  - *Do not consent to* access to your computer.
  - *Do not consent to* access to any documents you have in your possession.
- There is a difference between consent and a search warrant. *Never oppose a search warrant.*
- Do not make any statements to anyone, including:
  - Investigators
  - Coworkers
  - Managers or supervisors
- Keep in mind that statements made to management may be used against you just as surely as statements made to investigators.
- Keep silent until you are advised by an attorney.
- Keeping silent is especially important if you are innocent. Guilty people tend to manufacture lies that get them into trouble. Smart people talk to a lawyer.
- Your attorney must decide whether you wish to talk to the investigators or not.

- You are not compelled (and cannot lawfully be compelled) to talk to any investigator at any time unless the investigators grant you immunity, which would require legal advice anyway.
- Have your attorney arrange for any interview to be done at a time when that attorney can be present.
- Do not agree to speak to the investigator on their turf or on their terms. If they want to talk and your attorney believes it is a good idea, he or she can set it up at his or her office where the investigators do not have a home field advantage of being able to keep you confined and isolated.
- *Do not be unpleasant* when refusing to deal with investigators. Be professional. The government has attorneys, and you should have one too.
- *Do not destroy any documents*, even if you feel they are incriminating. Give them to your attorney.
- Do not make any written statements, and this means do not write a memo to the boss about the interaction because it could be admissible later.
- Do not make statements on behalf of your employer or produce documents on behalf of your employer without approval from your employer's general counsel.
- People usually talk themselves into prosecution, not out of it. *Silence is the best weapon an innocent person has.*
- If your attorney instructs you to give a statement or interview to authorities:
  - Make sure you *review all facts* before giving an interview or a statement.

- Make sure you understand every question before you answer it.
- *Always ask for clarification.*
- *Do not make assumptions.* Assumptions are always trouble.
- If you must assume a fact to answer a question, state the assumption in your answer.
- Answer only the questions asked.
- Do not volunteer information.
- *Do not speculate.*
- *Listen to your attorney.* Do not answer anything your attorney instructs you not to answer.

Wire Fraud and Mail Fraud

Caution: Under no circumstances should you act as your own attorney in defending criminal charges. If you or someone you know is accused of violating the following provisions you should:

1. Refuse to make any statements.
2. Obtain professional legal help from an experienced criminal lawyer immediately.

◼ Overview

18 USC § 1341: Elements of Mail and Wire Fraud

According to the U.S. Attorney's Manual there are two elements in mail fraud: (1) having devised or intending to devise a scheme to defraud (or to perform specified fraudulent acts), and (2) use of the mail for the purpose of executing, or attempting to execute, the scheme (or specified fraudulent acts). See *Schmuck v. United States*, 489 U.S. 705, 721 n. 10 (1989); *Pereira v. United States*, 347 U.S. 1, 8 (1954).

The elements of wire fraud under section 1343 directly parallel those of the mail fraud statute but require the use of an interstate telephone call or electronic communication made in furtherance of the scheme. See *United States v. Briscoe*, 65 F.3d 576, 583 (7th Cir. 1995) (citing *United States v. Ames Sintering Co.*, 927 F.2d 232, 234 [6th Cir.

1990] [per curiam]); *United States v. Frey,* 42 F.3d 795, 797 (3d Cir. 1994) (wire fraud is identical to the mail fraud statute except that it speaks of communications transmitted by wire); *United States v. Profit,* 49 F.3d 404, 406 n. 1 (8th Cir.).

Fortunately, the federal government does not prosecute mail or wire fraud if the scheme consists of isolated transactions between individuals involving minor loss to the victims. They do, however, prosecute schemes directed at defrauding a class of persons or the general public.

Mail and wire fraud in health care prosecutions involve health care companies using mail or wires to defraud patients or clients. For example:

- XYZ Home Care sends a bill to a patient that includes a $15 Medicare Cost Recovery Fee and implies that it is collecting this money because the government mandates it. If there is no such mandate, is XYZ committing mail fraud?
  - Yes, and if the bill is sent by fax, it is wire fraud.
- Is an e-mail message that falsely states information about a patient and sent to an insurance company mail fraud?
  - No, it is wire fraud. Electronic mail is not sent via the U.S. Postal Service or a similar delivery service (documents sent by Federal Express or UPS are considered the same as documents sent by the U.S. mail in terms of mail fraud). Because it is transmitted over the wires, it is considered wire fraud.

Prevention

The best insurance against a mail or wire fraud investigation is candor in all business dealings.

Legal First Aid

If someone from a federal or state investigative agency raises questions about mail fraud or wire fraud see "Legal First Aid: Read This First" in Chapter 8 on page 245.

Computer Fraud and Abuse Act 18 USC § 1030

Caution: Under no circumstances should you act as your own attorney in defending criminal charges. If you or someone you know is accused of violating the following provisions you should:

1. Refuse to make any statements.
2. Obtain professional legal help from an experienced criminal lawyer immediately.

■ Overview

The Computer Fraud and Abuse Act (CFAA) is a criminal statute that makes it a federal crime to "knowingly and with the intent to defraud, access a protected computer without authorization." It was originally designed to punish hackers for breaking into protected computer systems. A protected computer system is one that is used in interstate commerce. Because a hospital's computer system is used to send information back and forth to the federal and state governments and because it stores protected health care information, any intrusion into a hospital computer could be a violation of the CFAA.

Prevention

The surest way to prevent an issue under this statute is never to exceed an authorized use of the computer. If you have privileges in the computer system to see a certain category of information (all health care records) but only have privileges to alter a certain category of records (all respiratory care records), if you use another person's log-in information, or otherwise get into the system and perform tasks that you are not authorized to perform, you could be liable under the CFAA. For this reason, you never want to make unauthorized use of a computer at work. In addition to criminal penalties, there are civil penalties available to your employer in a separate lawsuit. For example:

- A nurse wants to see where Mr. Jones' wife is employed because she believes she knows her mother. She knows this information would be in the hospital financial records. She gets a user name and password from a friend in Patient Accounts and looks this information up. Has she violated the CFAA?

  - Under a strict reading of the statute, she has violated the CFAA. The nurse could be liable for civil and criminal penalties.

- A respiratory therapist employed part time as a home care therapist for a Durable Medical Equipment company wants to get a list of all the patients who have home oxygen. He knows he can get a pretty good idea by looking at the computer in the pulmonary function laboratory and reading the test results of these patients. He then uses this information to help his home care company get patients for home oxygen therapy. Has he violated the CFAA?

  - He may not have violated the CFAA because the hospital pulmonary function computer was not used in interstate commerce or to transmit data across the wires.

However, he may still be liable under HIPAA for a privacy violation.

Legal First Aid

If someone from a federal or state investigative agency raises questions about any unauthorized use of a computer, see "Legal First Aid: Read This First" on page 245.

False Statements to Investigators

Caution: Under no circumstances should you act as your own attorney in defending criminal charges. If you or someone you know is accused of violating the following provisions you should:
1. Refuse to make any statements.
2. Obtain professional legal help from an experienced criminal lawyer immediately.

▇ Overview
If you follow the advice in this book, you do not need to worry about this section. If you do not make statements to investigators, you do not have to worry about this section. So, at the risk of saying it again, do not give a statement to any investigator without your attorney present and only then if the attorney advises you to do so. If you do give a statement, it must be completely truthful.

False Statements to a Federal Investigator
The circumstance often arises in which a false statement is made voluntarily or in response to an inquiry by an FBI or other federal agent. 18 USC § 1001 penalizes this conduct.

It is the government's policy not to charge a violation in situations in which a suspect, during an investigation, merely denies guilt in response to questioning by the government. This policy is narrowly construed, however; affirmative, voluntary statements to federal criminal investigators that are knowingly false do not fall within the policy.

By its plain terms, § 1001 (as it existed before it was amended in October 1996) broadly reaches "[w]hoever, in any matter within the jurisdiction of any department or agency of the United States knowingly and willfully . . . makes any false, fictitious or fraudulent statements or representations. . . ."

For example, if the false statement was volunteered to an FBI agent the Supreme Court has held that § 1001 does apply. See *United States v. Rodgers*, 466 U.S. 475 (1984). In *Rodgers* the court concluded the following: (1) that criminal investigations fell within the term "in any matter" and (2) that the FBI qualified as a "department or agency." In *Rodgers* the language "within the jurisdiction" was held to merely differentiate the official, authorized functions of an agency or department from matters peripheral to the business of that body.

Although § 1001 does not provide for exceptions, a number of courts have held that it does not apply to cases involving simple false denials of guilt in response to government initiated inquiries. See *United States v. Taylor*, 907 F.2d 801 (8th Cir. 1990); *United States v. Equihua-Juarez*, 851 F.2d 1222 (9th Cir. 1988);

Other courts have rejected the "exculpatory no" exception to § 1001. See *United States v. Rodriguez-Rios*, 14 F.3d 1040 (5th Cir. 1994) (en banc).

For example:

- An FBI agent investigating John Smith goes to see Jane Doe at the offices of XYZ Home Care. The FBI agent wants to know if John Smith worked on May 1. Jane knows that John did not

work on that date but says, "yes, he worked."
Because the FBI agent is not investigating
Jane, is she in any trouble?

- Yes. She made a knowingly false statement
to the FBI.

Prevention

The best prevention against a false statements
prosecution is not to make any statements about
anything until you have legal representation. Even
if you misstate the facts out of ignorance or mistake, the federal government may still claim you
had an intention to mislead investigators. For this
reason the only thing that prevents this kind of
prosecution is silence.

Legal First Aid

If someone from a federal or state investigative
agency starts to ask questions about any criminal
matter, see "Legal First Aid: Read This First" on
page 245.

False Claims

Caution: Under no circumstances should you act as your own attorney in defending criminal charges. If you or someone you know is accused of violating the following provisions you should:

1. Refuse to make any statements.
2. Obtain professional legal help from an experienced criminal lawyer immediately.

■ Overview

A false claim is a false demand for payment made to the United States (or the failure to refund a payment made under a mistake of fact). Normally, these arise in health care in connection with billing programs that are aimed at maximizing revenue. Normally, the health care worker who provides clinical services is a fact witness only in these matters, but there have been frequent prosecutions of physicians who have stepped over the line and made false bills to the United States.

Statutes

Although Congress has enacted numerous specific statutes to deal with particular types of fraud against the government, enforcement efforts rely on five general statutes: 18 USC §§ 287 (false claims), 371 (conspiracy), 1001 (false statements),

1341 (mail fraud), and 1343 (wire fraud). The mail fraud and wire fraud statutes (18 USC §§ 1341, 1343) are discussed above in the first section of this chapter; the other statutes are discussed here.

Title 18 U.S. Code § 287—the false claims statute—provides in part as follows:

> Whoever makes or presents to any person or officer in the civil, military or naval service of the United States, or to any department or agency thereof, any claim upon or against the United States, or any department or agency thereof, knowing such claim to be false, fictitious, or fraudulent, shall be imprisoned not more than five years.

There is also a companion conspiracy statute, 18 USC § 286. In 1863 Congress enacted a false claims and statements statute "in the wake of a spate of frauds upon the government." See *United States v. Bramblett*, 348 U.S. 503, 504 (1955). As originally enacted the statute penalized presentment "for payment or approval of false claims upon or against the Government" (*Bramblett*, 348 U.S. at 504) as well as false statements made "for the purpose of obtaining, or aiding in obtaining, the approval or payment of such claim." On June 25, 1948, the statute was divided into 18 USC § 287 and 18 USC § 1001, respectively (62 Stat. 749)

The § 287 statute is designed to "protect the government against those who would cheat or mislead it in the administration of its programs" (*United States v. White*, 27 F 3d 1531, 1535 [11th Cir. 1094]), and it has been used to combat fraudulent claims filed under numerous federal programs, including Medicare and Medicaid. White (Medicare claims by a chiropractor); *United States v. Hooshmand*, 931 F.2d 725, 733 (11th Cir. 1991) (Medicare claims for tests).

For example:

- A physician codes all patient visits as being "extensive" and charges Medicare the extended office visit price even though he often spends less than 10 minutes with these patients. If he actually spent 45 minutes with each patient based on the number of patients seen in a given day, he would have worked 29 hours every day. Is this a false claim?

  - Yes. It may also be wire fraud and mail fraud.

Prevention

The best prevention against a false claim is strict honesty in billing. Providers who look for an angle to increase their revenue and believe they will not get caught usually overlook 31 USC § 3729, which provides a financial incentive to whistle-blowers to let the government know about the fraud.

Legal First Aid

If someone from a federal or state investigative agency starts to ask questions about any criminal matter, see "Legal First Aid: Read This First" on page 245.

HIPAA

Caution: Under no circumstances should you act as your own attorney in defending criminal charges. If you or someone you know is accused of violating the following provisions you should:

1. Refuse to make any statements.
2. Obtain professional legal help from an experienced criminal lawyer immediately.

Overview

The Health Insurance Portability and Accountability Act (HIPAA) is the federal privacy statute. It is designed to prevent individuals without authorization from gaining access to protected health information. The purpose behind the rule is to prevent Medicare and insurance fraud as well as to prevent identity theft. To date there have been relatively few successful prosecutions for violations of HIPAA, and the federal government does not have an official policy in writing that details for the government how it will handle these cases. The Justice Department has suggested in memoranda that it would go after employers for the acts of employees in sharing protected health information. Most cases, to date, have involved private litigation, not criminal litigation. However, there are criminal penalties built into the HIPAA statute.

A former cancer center employee was the first to plead guilty to criminal violation of the privacy-related provisions of HIPAA, P.L. 104-191. The guilty plea represents the first ever criminal conviction under the privacy statute. Importantly, the employee was not a "covered entity" as required under the statute, and some legal analysts believe this signals an intent to pursue more criminal matters even though HIPAA arguably does not apply directly to individuals.

The U.S. Attorney in Washington state charged the employee under 42 USC § 1320d-6(a)(3) and (b)(3) providing that a person who knowingly, and in violation of HIPAA, discloses individually identifiable health information to another person with intent to "sell, transfer, or use individually identifiable health information for commercial advantage, personal gain, or malicious harm," may be fined not more than $250,000, imprisoned not more than 10 years, or both. Because the defendant pleaded he was due to be sentenced to only 10 to 16 months in federal prison.

For example:

- Your cousin Bob has a flower delivery service. He wants to know the names of patients admitted to the hospital so that he can call and offer to deliver flowers to their rooms. You provide it to him. Did you violate HIPAA?
  - Yes. If you are a covered entity or employed by a covered entity, you cannot disclose patient information.

Prevention

The best prevention against a HIPAA claim is to never under any circumstances, even to help out friends or relatives, divulge protected health information to anyone.

Legal First Aid

If someone from a federal or state investigative agency starts to ask questions about access to medical records, see "Legal First Aid: Read This First" for criminal law matters on page 245.

Financial Crimes

Caution: Under no circumstances should you act as your own attorney in defending criminal charges. If you or someone you know is accused of violating the following provisions you should:

1. Refuse to make any statements.
2. Obtain professional legal help from an experienced criminal lawyer immediately.

Overview

Federal financial crimes in health care usually occur in two ways: (1) theft of money or property from patients under circumstances that violate federal laws and (2) theft of credit cards or personal information from patients for use in identity theft. In either situation there is almost no hope of getting away with this kind of theft. Credit card transactions at stores like Wal-Mart are videotaped. ATM machines usually feature video surveillance. Patients usually remember how much money they brought with them to the hospital. Under no circumstances should you ever be foolish enough to believe you could get away with theft. Identity theft is a high priority among federal law enforcers. Again, even dabbling at this (e.g., collecting social security numbers) is playing with fire.

Sometimes, however, patients do misidentify people who they believe took money or property. In that situation you need to hire an attorney and defend yourself.

Prevention

The first step in prevention is to develop a good bond with patients and a good reputation for honesty. Most of us have this and do this naturally. It is a good idea to keep assignment sheets and other data that show what rooms and assignments you had for a couple of days to prove where you were and what you did if an issue ever arises about the loss or theft of personal property.

Legal First Aid

If someone from a federal or state investigative agency starts to ask questions about theft of patient information or other financial crimes, see "Legal First Aid: Read This First" for criminal law matters on page 245.

Federal Anti-Kickback Statute

Caution: Under no circumstances should you act as your own attorney in defending criminal charges. If you or someone you know is accused of violating the following provisions you should:
1. Refuse to make any statements.
2. Obtain professional legal help from an experienced criminal lawyer immediately.

▉ Overview

The Medicare and Medicaid Patient Protection Act of 1987, as amended, 42 USC §1320a-7b (the "Anti-Kickback Statute"), establishes criminal penalties for paying or receiving compensation in connection with referrals to Medicare and state health care (e.g., Medicaid) insurance plans.

Section 1320a-7b(b) provides as follows:

(1) whoever knowingly and willfully solicits or receives any remuneration (including any kickback, bribe or rebate) directly or indirectly, overtly or covertly, in cash or in kind - (A) in return for referring an individual to a person for the furnishing or arranging for the furnishing of any item or service for which payment may be made in whole or in part under [Medicare] or a State health care program, or (B) in return for purchasing, leasing, ordering, or arranging for or recommending purchasing,

leasing, or ordering any good, facility, service, or item for which payment may be made in whole or in part under [Medicare] or a State health care program, shall be guilty of a felony and upon conviction thereof, shall be fined not more than $25,000 or imprisoned for not more than five years, or both.

The law not only makes it a crime to solicit or receive any compensation or remuneration, it also criminalizes paying such compensation:

(2) whoever knowingly and willfully offers and pays any remuneration (including any kickback, bribe or rebate) directly or indirectly, overtly or covertly, in cash or in kind to any person to induce such person - (A) to refer an individual to a person for the furnishing or arranging for the furnishing of any item or service for which payment may be made in whole or in part under [Medicare] or a State health care program, or (B) to purchase, lease, order, or arrange for or recommend purchasing, leasing, or ordering any good, facility, service, or item for which payment may be made in whole or in part under [Medicare] or a State health care program, shall be guilty of a felony and upon conviction thereof, shall be fined not more than $25,000 or imprisoned for not more than five years, or both.

The anti-kickback law prevents a person from asking for, receiving, or paying any type of kickback, bribe, gratuity, or remuneration, whether it is in cash or in kind (e.g., deep discounts, free services), in exchange for referring patients under Medicare or Medicaid.

There are certain "safe harbors" that the Office of Inspector General for the Department of Health and Human Services has spelled out in regulations. Those are beyond the scope of this section.

For example:

- XYZ Home Care wants to get more referrals from ABC Hospital. It asks the Director of Physical Therapy at ABC Hospital to do a quarterly inservice for its staff on home care aids for which it will pay him $500. The Director of Physical Therapy sends several patients to XYZ over the next few months. He had never recommended their services previously. If the Director of Physical Therapy provides the inservices he gets a check. If he fails to provide the inservices, he still gets a check. Is this a violation?
  - Yes. The object of the relationship to a neutral third party would lead to the conclusion that the payments are not for education but to induce referrals. Both XYZ and the Director could be criminally charged.

Prevention

If you desire to compensate or seek compensation for services and you believe that at least some part of that arrangement has some relationship to the care of patients who receive payment for their services by Medicare or Medicaid, then you must seek a legal opinion before entering into the relationship. Even if the principal purpose of the relationship is not to induce referrals, if there is an inducement of any kind, it violates this statute and can result in criminal prosecution and sometimes civil monetary penalties on top of false claims.

Legal First Aid

If someone from a federal or state investigative agency raises questions about your payment or referral practices, see "Legal First Aid: Read This First" for criminal law matters on page 245.

doctor is in charge and makes all medical decisions in the case and has decided not to make a report, can the therapist rely on the doctor and legally fail to make a report?

- No, the responsibility is individual, and the therapist must make a report.

Prevention

The best prevention against a prosecution for failure to report abuse is to report any abuse you see or suspect. Even if the elder simply has very frail skin and the bruises are a result of drug therapy, this is not a determination for the individual health care worker. Even if the elder denies abuse (this is common), the report should be made. Investigators will be assigned to determine if there was abuse.

Legal First Aid

If someone from a federal or state investigative agency starts to ask questions about any criminal matter, see "Legal First Aid: Read This First" on page 245.

Resources

- International Network for the Prevention of Elder Abuse and information on World Elder Abuse Awareness Day (available online at http://www.inpea.net).
- National Center on Elder Abuse—data, fact sheets, and other information on elder abuse, neglect, and exploitation in the United States (available online at http://www.ncea.aoa.gov).
- The National Clearinghouse on Abuse in Later Life—information on coordinating elder abuse prevention efforts with domestic violence and sexual assault programs (available online at http://www.ncall.us).

- Contact your local area agency for information about volunteering to call or visit an isolated senior.
- Eldercare Locator (available online at http://www.eldercare.gov).
- See Appendix 5 for a list of elder abuse hotlines.

Child Abuse

Caution: Under no circumstances should you act as your own attorney in defending criminal charges. If you or someone you know is accused of violating the following provisions you should:

1. Refuse to make any statements.
2. Obtain professional legal help from an experienced criminal lawyer immediately.

■ Overview

Child abuse can take many forms, but the most common is physical abuse directed at a child. It is most often accompanied by a parent who professes no knowledge (or specious knowledge) of the injury. Often, there is a boyfriend or a step-parent who is the abuser and who has significant control over the parent of the child. These are very difficult situations. In nearly every state a health care worker is a mandatory reporter and must report any suspicion of child abuse to authorities.

Who Must Report Child Abuse?

- *Private citizen reporters:* Any citizen may (and should) report child abuse, but the failure to do so is not a crime. Covering up the abuse or lying to investigators is. In most states all reports are confidential, and citizens who are not required to report the abuse are not even required to give their names. They are also protected from civil and criminal liability as long as they make the report of child abuse in good faith.

- *Mandated reporters:* All employees, serving in any capacity, in health care (nurses, physicians, therapists, and aides) and education (school nurses, counselors, teachers, and principals). Law enforcement officers are also mandatory reporters. In addition, in some states a person who has assumed responsibility for the care or custody of a child (for example, a daycare worker), even if they are not being paid for the service, is also considered a mandated reporter.

Duty to Report

All statutorily mandated reporters must report actual or suspected abuse. The reporting responsibility is individual for each mandated reporter. Failure to report the abuse if a reasonable person would have believed the injuries were sustained through abuse could result in prosecution in nearly every state. Although the case law and the results of cases vary from state to state, the law requires that abuse be reported, and the failure to report abuse can result in civil and criminal sanctions.

How to Make an Abuse Report

- Call the state hotline (see Appendix 6).
- Make the report immediately or as soon as possible by telephone.
  For example:
- A respiratory therapist finds a 6-year-old boy with multiple small burns over his arms, chest, and back while providing a treatment in the